Proteinuria

Proteinuria

Edited by
M. M. Avram
The Long Island College Hospital
Brooklyn, New York

PLENUM MEDICAL BOOK COMPANY
New York and London

Library of Congress Cataloging in Publication Data

Main entry under title:

Proteinuria.

Includes bibliographies and index.
1. Proteinuria. 2. Kidney—Disease—Diagnosis. I. Avram, Morrell M. (Morrell
Michael), 1929–   . [DNLM: 1. Proteinuria. WJ 343 P967]
RC905.P76   1985   616.6′1   85-9305
ISBN-13: 978-1-4612-9502-0   e-ISBN-13: 978-1-4613-2477-5
DOI: 10.1007/978-1-4613-2477-5

© 1985 Plenum Publishing Corporation
Softcover reprint of the hardcover 1st edition 1985
233 Spring Street, New York, N.Y. 10013

Plenum Medical Book Company is an imprint of Plenum Publishing Corporation

To Maria, Rella, Marc, Eric, Mathew,
and David with admiration
for their relentless will,
idealism, and hard work

Contributors

A. J. ADLER, M.D., Chief, Home Dialysis, Associate Professor of Medicine, V. A. Hospital, Brooklyn, New York

M. M. AVRAM, M.D., Chief, Division of Nephrology, Medical Director, The Avram Center for Kidney Diseases, The Long Island College Hospital, Clinical Professor of Medicine, Department of Medicine, Downstate Medical Center, Medical Director, Brooklyn Kidney Center and Nephrology Foundation of Brooklyn, Brooklyn, New York

DAVID S. BALDWIN, M.D., Professor of Medicine, Department of Medicine, New York University Medical Center, New York, New York

G. M. BERLYNE, M.D., Professor of Medicine, Department of Medicine, Downstate Medical Center, Chief, Nephrology Section, V.A. Hospital, Brooklyn, New York

JOHN D. BOWER, M.D., Professor of Medicine, Department of Medicine, University of Mississippi Medical Center, Director, Artificial Kidney Unit, Medical Director, Kidney Care, Inc., Jackson, Mississippi

BARRY M. BRENNER, M.D., Samuel A. Levine Professor of Medicine, Department of Medicine, Harvard Medical School, Director, Renal Division, Brigham & Women's Hospital, Boston, Massachusetts

D. E. BROWN, M.D., Instructor, Department of Medicine, V. A. Hospital, Brooklyn, New York

KHALID M. H. BUTT, M.D., Associate Professor of Surgery, Downstate Medical Center, Brooklyn, New York

MARIA JOSE F. CAMARGO, Research Associate, Department of Physiology, Cornell University Medical College, New York, New York

GAY CASE, R.N., Home Training Unit, Kidney Care, Inc., University of Mississippi Medical Center, Jackson, Mississippi

JHOONG S. CHEIGH, M.D., Director, Inpatient Services, Assistant Professor of Medicine, Cornell University Medical Center, New York, New York

PAUL D. DOOLAN, M.D., Professor of Medicine, Department of Medicine, Yale University Medical Center, Division of Nephrology, St. Mary's Hospital, Waterbury, Connecticut

LANCE D. DWORKIN, M.D., Assistant Professor of Medicine, Department of Medicine, N.Y.U. Medical Center, New York, New York

PIERRE F. FAUBERT, M.D., Assistant Professor of Medicine, Department of Medicine, Downstate Medical Center, Attending, Division of Nephrology, Brookdale Hospital and Medical Center, Brooklyn, New York

ELI A. FRIEDMAN, M.D., Professor of Medicine, Department of Medicine, Chief, Renal Diseases Division, Downstate Medical Center, Brooklyn, New York

RICHARD J. GLASSOCK, M.D., Professor and Chairman, Department of Medicine, Harbor U.C.L.A. Medical Center, Torrance, California

CYRIL J. GODEC, M.D., Director, Department of Urology, The Long Island College Hospital, Brooklyn, New York

JOHN P. HAYSLETT, M.D., Professor of Medicine, Department of Medicine, Chief, Section of Nephrology, Yale University School of Medicine, New Haven, Connecticut

JOHN E. KILEY, M.D., Professor in Medicine & Nephrology, The University of Mississippi Medical Center, Jackson, Mississippi

JAMES M. LUCIANO, M.D., Resident, Department of Medicine, Downstate Medical Center, State University of New York, Brooklyn, New York

THOMAS MAACK, M.D., Professor of Physiology, Cornell University Medical College, New York, New York

JOHN F. MAHER, M.D., Professor of Medicine, Department of Medicine, Director, Nephrology Division, Uniformed Services University of the Health Sciences School of Medicine, Bethesda, Maryland

ARAM V. MANOUKIAN, M.D., Senior Medical Student, Department of Medicine, Downstate Medical Center, State University of New York, Brooklyn, New York

ILENE MILLER, M.D., Instructor in Medicine, Department of Medicine, Assistant Attending Physician, Department of Medicine, Cornell University Medical Center, New York, New York

JANET MOURADIAN, M.D., Clinical Professor of Pathology, Cornell University Medical Center, New York, New York

BRYAN D. MYERS, M.D., Associate Professor of Medicine, Department of Medicine, Division of Nephrology, Stanford University School of Medicine, Stanford, California

C. HYUNG PARK, M.D., Research Associate, Department of Physiology, Cornell University Medical College, New York, New York

JEROME G. PORUSH, M.D., Chief, Division of Nephrology, Brookdale Hospital Medical Center, Professor of Medicine, Department of Medicine, Downstate Medical Center, Brooklyn, New York

ROSCOE R. ROBINSON, M.D., Vice Chancellor, Medical Affairs, Vanderbilt University Medical Center, Professor of Medicine, Department of Medicine, Vanderbilt University Medical Center, Nashville, Tennessee

J. E. RUBIN, M.D., Chief, Hemodialysis, V. A. Hospital, Brooklyn, New York

GEORGE E. SCHREINER, M.D., Director, Nephrology Division, Professor of Medicine, Department of Medicine, Georgetown University School of Medicine, Washington, D.C.

M. SEIDMAN, M.D., Attending Physician, Department of Medicine, Nephrology Section, V. A. Hospital, Assistant Professor of Medicine, Department of Medicine, Downstate Medical Center, Brooklyn, New York

KURT H. STENZEL, M.D., Medical Director, Rogosin Kidney Center, Professor of Medicine, Biochemistry & Surgery, Chief, Division of Nephrology, The New York Hospital—Cornell Medical Center, New York, New York

J. SUTTON, M.D., Instructor, Department of Medicine, V. A. Hospital, Brooklyn, New York

JOHN WANG, M.D., Department of Medicine, Cornell University Medical Center, New York, New York

Preface

Decoding the significance of proteinuria as an indicator of severity or prognosis in kidney disease is a stimulating challenge to students and practitioners of nephrology. Sir Richard Bright in 1827 associated proteinuria with the disease that bears his name. In the subsequent more than a century and a half, however, the meaning of the linkage between proteinuria and renal disease remains elusive.

Proteinuria is discovered on routine urinalysis in about 10 million Americans, most of whom express no symptoms of kidney disease, each year. From the studies of Robinson (updated in these pages), we know that proteinuria, *per se*, can be present for 20 years without change in renal function, as described in orthostatic proteinuria. By contrast, proteinuria may be the harbinger of swift kidney destruction, rarely culminating in clinical collapse, a syndrome typifying "malignant proteinuria" as detailed herein by Avram.

Although proteinuria is ubiquitous, an orderly management strategy for rational handling of proteinuria of less than nephrotic range is lacking. Separation of tubular proteinuria and transient proteinuria of fever is now possible routinely. This book provides a record of the contributions of investigators and clinicians whose work forms the substrate for production of understanding and, ultimately, marching orders for practitioners seeking optimized management for their proteinuric patients.

Generations of investigators have attempted to connect specific urinary proteins with distinct kidney disorders. This feat was the result of serendipity in the 1950 observation that Bence Jones proteins are present in most patients with multiple myeloma. Over the ensuing 20 years, it was learned that small amounts of Bence Jones protein may be present in normal urine and, more importantly, that the careful study of these urinary constituents and their precursors would serve as a Rosetta stone for clarification of modern immunology.

Might we repeat the successes of the multiple myeloma story by readdressing superficially simple questions? What is proteinuria? What does its presence mean? And how does its presence alter the biology of the patient or the function of the kidney? Despite its high prevalence, we do not know whether proteinuria is injurious to the kidney or is the product of renal damage, nor do we know (with limited exceptions such as the proteinuria of diabetes or uncontrolled hypertension) how to prevent or whether and in what way to treat it.

Until the significance to the patient of documenting proteinuria is elucidated, it will continue as an underdetected and inadequately studied mark of kidney disease. As our society reappraises health care costs, including billions spent on the treatment of renal insufficiency, it is appropriate to direct energy and resources in an attempt to prevent renal disease. Toward this goal, the Division of Nephrology's Avram Center for Kidney Diseases of The Long Island College Hospital in Brooklyn assembled these manuscripts on "Proteinuria." It is the editor's hope that this volume will convey the excitement and enthusiasm of the authors. It is the wish of all who contributed that the new information developed may benefit the many patients found to have proteinuria.

This book is divided to consider first a description of proteinuria and its relationship to glomerular and tubular functions. Subsequently, the clinical consequences and management of proteinuria are reviewed. A unique variety of renal protein loss termed "malignant proteinuria" is described, along with its management by pharmacological functional desctruction of the kidneys, a desperate therapeutic maneuver for desperately ill patients, which is euphemistically called medical nephrectomy.

In this tome, representing contributions by brilliant researchers from our prestigious national universities from coast to coast, we take a step in the direction of finding needed answers for the millions of Americans who have proteinuria. Converting tens of years of work by my colleagues and me into a synthesis of the state of the art of proteinuria research has been a fulfilling labor of joy.

M. M. Avram, M.D.

Acknowledgments

We wish to acknowledge the support of the National Kidney Foundation of New York, the Avram Center for Kidney Diseases of The Long Island College Hospital, and The Long Island College Hospital.

Special thanks to Ms. Phyllis LeBeau for invaluable editorial and technical assistance.

Contents

Part I. Mechanisms of Proteinuria

Part II. Clinical Expressions of Proteinuria

Part I

Mechanisms of Proteinuria

A good story has a beginning, middle, and end. Proteinuria begins in the glomerulus. Its origin, formerly a mystery, is now recognized as the result of forces impinging on both sides of the glomerular membrane.

Brenner and Dworkin dissect these forces in an analysis of what is now known as glomerular permselectivity. Extrapolating from masterful experiments in the rat employing dextran and other macromolecules as probes, these investigators were able to change glomerular protein selectivity by altering electrical charge and thus molecular configuration at the capillary wall of the glomerulus. It is inferred by Brenner and Dworkin that, in health, the negatively charged glomerular capillary wall acts as a barrier to filtration of plasma protein and other macromolecules while permitting a high ratio of fluid filtration. Although the exact anatomic location of the barrier to transglomerular passage of macromolecules is unknown, the negative endothelial charge probably inhibits passage of polyanions. Neutral macromolecules are impeded by the basement membrane, and cationic solutes are barred by epithelial slit diaphragms.

Myers, a student of Brenner, extended the use of dextran probes to 20 healthy humans who were given infusions of uncharged dextran to characterize molecular sieving factors. Because naturally occurring proteins in serum undergo tubular reabsorption, they are unsuitable to test the glomerular filtration barrier. However, dextran, a nonprotein polymer of D-glucopyranose, is neither excreted nor reabsorbed by the tubule and tests well the glomerular membrane barrier. Myers's results validate his mentor's original observations in the rat and show that in the human, solute charge, size, and molecular configuration are important determinants of passage across the glomerular barrier, as are biophysical factors such as driving pressure and oncotic pressure. In an original exploration of the mechanism of protein leakage in the nephrotic syndrome, Myers's results in 70 patients with nephrotic range pro-

1

teinuria sustain the conclusion that protein enters the nephron because of an alteration of membrane pore structure.

Loss of size selectivity, he suggests, rather than charge selectivity is the cause of massive (and, rarely, malignant) proteinuria. It may be predicted that application of neutral and charged macromolecular probes to the study of various nephropathies (already underway in diabetes) will be a major means of improving understanding of proteinuria.

Maack and associates tackle the complex task of determining how the renal tubule handles protein using albumin as a marker in isolated, perfused rabbit proximal tubules. This comprehensive manuscript suggests that tubular absorption and catabolism of proteins, as exemplified by albumin, may intensify the severity of some forms of the nephrotic syndrome. It also echoes a seminal finding of Jean Oliver, who, while working for five decades at The Long Island College Hospital, was the first to understand and report that "hyaline droplets" in renal cells of nephrotic kidneys were evidence for protein absorption.

Tubular pathology, long neglected because of more obvious morphological alterations in glomeruli, may be about to assume center stage in what is probably the middle of the drama of unraveling renal pathophysiology. Maher lists and reviews the diseases that cause tubular proteinuria. Tubular proteinuria, he believes, is a manifestation that can be used to group some renal diseases (e.g., analgesic nephropathies, multiple myeloma, methicillin coma, transplant rejection) that may differ in pathogenesis from other kidney disorders. The role of hypercalcemia and hyperparathyroidism as aggravating factors in the genesis of tubular (interstitial) nephropathies is reviewed.

Robinson, in an ongoing study unique to nephrology, weighs the significance of isolated proteinuria in otherwise normal individuals. These elegant studies span a follow-up period of over 20 years. This report emphasizes the importance of the patterns of proteinuria, with "constant" proteinuria more likely to be associated with clinical renal disease than is the "intermittent" type. Orthostatic proteinuria cannot be regarded as absolutely benign, since in at least some cases it may reflect incipient kidney disease. Kidney biopsy reading from young men with fixed orthostatic proteinuria revealed that 8% had glomerular pathology on light microscopy. On the positive side, however, neither renal disease nor reduced kidney function were observed after the "first" 20 years of Robinson's intellectual inquiry, unique in the annals of nephrology.

M.M.A.

1

Glomerular Permselectivity

BARRY M. BRENNER and LANCE D. DWORKIN

GLOMERULAR FILTRATION OF MACROMOLECULES

The process of glomerular filtration results in the separation of approximately one-fifth to one-third of the plasma entering the glomeruli of each kidney into a solution that has the characteristics of a nearly ideal ultrafiltrate. This high rate of fluid filtration is driven by the hydraulic force created by the pumping action of the heart. However, despite the extremely low resistance of this capillary wall to the flux of water, this same structure normally impedes the filtration of circulating macromolecules (substances with molecular weights of several thousand or more), so that the concentrations of all but the smallest plasma proteins in the glomerular ultrafiltrate are exceedingly small.

In recent years, the permeability characteristics of the glomerular capillary wall have been examined by both ultrastructural and differential clearance techniques. As a result of these studies, several factors that determine the glomerular filtration of macromolecules have been identified, including molecular size, molecular charge, molecular configuration, and glomerular hemodynamics. This discussion considers the mechanisms whereby these factors influence the filtration of macromolecules.

SIZE SELECTIVITY OF THE GLOMERULAR CAPILLARY WALL

Clearance techniques have been utilized to study the glomerular filtration of macromolecules *in vivo* on both man and animals. Such

BARRY M. BRENNER • Laboratory of Kidney and Electrolyte Physiology, Department of Medicine, Harvard Medical School; Renal Division, Brigham & Women's Hospital, Boston, Massachusetts 02115.   LANCE D. DWORKIN • Department of Medicine, New York University Medical Center, New York, New York 10016.

studies have generally employed a single macromolecular species, such as dextran, as the test solute. Dextrans are useful because they are homogeneous in chemical structure, molecular configuration, and molecular charge, but their molecular weights, and therefore size, can be intentionally varied over a wide range of values. If a test macromolecule (M), such as dextran, is neither secreted nor reabsorbed by the renal tubules, then a measure of the glomerular filtration of M is provided by the ratio of the clearance of M to the clearance of inulin. This clearance ratio, known as the fractional clearance of M, will be equal to the Bowman's space-to-plasma concentration ratio of M.

Dextrans and a variety of dextran derivatives have been demonstrated to satisfy the requirement that their rate of excretion equal their rate of filtration (no net secretion or reabsorption occurs), and thus the fractional clearance of dextran becomes a convenient measure of permselectivity, varying from zero when dextran molecules are impermeant to 1 when molecules are as freely permeable as inulin.[1-3] Fig. 1 (left) shows the effects of increasing molecular size on the fractional clearance of uncharged tritiated dextrans (solid circles) across the glomerular capillary walls of normal Munich–Wistar rats.[3] Fractional clearance is plotted as a function of effective dextran radius, the latter determined by gel chromatographic techniques.[3] A value of 1 on the ordinate corresponds to a neutral dextran clearance equal to that of inulin. It can be seen from Fig. 1 that, on average, measurable restriction to filtration of neutral dextran (fractional clearances less than 1) does not occur until effective dextran radii exceed approximately 20 Å. Beyond that radius, mean fractional clearances decrease progressively with increasing molecular size, approaching zero at radii of about 42 Å or greater. Similar values have been obtained in other studies of dog, man, and other strains of rat using dextrans as well as polyvinylpyrrolidone, another neutral polymer.[4-10]

THEORY OF RESTRICTED TRANSPORT THROUGH PORES

Pappenheimer and co-workers[11,12] first applied hydrodynamic models of solute transport through pores to capillaries. As applied to the glomerular capillary, this model envisions transport of solute as taking place through large numbers of identical cylindrical pores. Macromolecular solutes are postulated to behave as solid spheres moving in a fluid continuum. Using this approximation, one can compute the hindrances such solutes encounter in moving through the pores by solving the hydrodynamic equations that describe the slow motion of a sphere

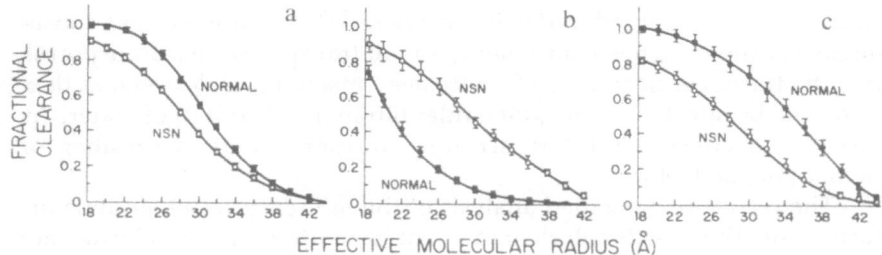

EFFECTIVE MOLECULAR RADIUS (Å)

Figure 1. Fractional clearances of neutral dextrans (left), anionic dextran sulfates (middle), and cationic diethylaminoethyl (DEAE) dextrans (right) plotted as functions of effective molecular radii for normal rats and those with nephrotoxic serum nephritis (NSN) [Data (mean ± S.E.) from references 1–3]. (Reprinted with permission from Brenner et al.[48])

through a fluid-filled tube. For uncharged spherical molecules, such solute–membrane interactions depend only on the ratio of the solute molecular radius to pore radius (λ).[13] The solute flux approaches zero as the solute size nears the pore size ($\lambda \to 1$), and, conversely, solute movement is unhindered if the pore is very large ($\lambda \to 0$). A rigorous presentation of the mathematical formalism underlying pore theory is given elsewhere.[14,15]

Using fractional neutral dextran clearance data together with simultaneously measured values for the determinants of single-nephron glomerular filtration rate (SNGFR) in the normal rat, Chang and associates[3,16] were able to calculate a particular value for λ for each dextran radius. A measure of the utility of pore theory as a model of solute transport across the glomerular wall is provided by the degree to which computed values for pore radius are found to be independent of molecular size, as all molecules presumably traverse the same size pores. Over the range of dextran studied, Chang et al.[3,16] found that a pore radius of about 50 Å fits well with the data in the Munich–Wistar rat. Similar average values have also been reported for the glomerular capillaries of dogs[5,10] and humans.[4] Thus, in terms of size selectivity, the normal glomerular capillary wall acts as a membrane with uniform pores of 50 Å radius.

HEMODYNAMIC DETERMINANTS OF THE TRANSPORT OF MACROMOLECULES

It is important to recognize that the transport of macromolecules across the glomerular capillary wall is not only a function of molecular

size. Thus, as discussed in detail elsewhere,[3,13,16,17] an important consequence of the diffusive component of total transglomerular transport is
that the fractional clearances of "diffusive" macromolecules such as dextrans will be affected by the glomerular filtration rate (GFR) of water. As
already discussed, GFR is strongly influenced by a number of
hemodynamic factors.

The results of a detailed analysis of the influences of hemodynamic
factors on the fractional clearances of a neutral macromolecule are
presented in Fig. 2.[16] This figure depicts the theoretical effects on macromolecular transport of selective perturbations in the four determinants
of ultrafiltration, namely, initial glomerular plasma flow rate, Q_A, mean
transcapillary hydraulic pressure difference, $\overline{\Delta P}$, initial glomerular capillary plasma protein concentration, C_A, and the ultrafiltration coefficient,
K_f. Theoretical fractional clearance values for a homologous series of
neutral macromolecules (M), C_M/C_{IN}, are plotted as a function of the effective hydrodynamic radius of M in each panel, based on input quantities representative of the normal Munich–Wistar rat. Once again, M is
assumed to be excreted at a rate that equals its filtration, so that C_M/C_{IN}
is equivalent to the concentration ratio of M in Bowman's space to
plasma water. Panel A in Fig. 2 depicts the alterations in the fractional
clearance of M expected to follow variations in Q_A. Here, the middle
curve corresponds to a value of Q_A of 75 nl/min, the usual value observed in the Munich–Wistar rat under conditions of normal hydrope-
nia. Since, as discussed above, GFR and SNGFR are highly plasma-flow
dependent in this species, increases in Q_A are expected to increase volume flux more than solute flux, so that the ratio C_M/C_{IN} will decline. Importantly, even though the fractional clearance of M declines, the absolute clearance of M is expected to increase, but to a lesser extent than
the corresponding clearance of water as determined by C_{IN}. Of course,
a decline in Q_A will have the opposite effect.

The effects of variations in the mean net hydraulic pressure differ-
ence, $\overline{\Delta P}$, are shown in Fig. 2B. Declines in the value of $\overline{\Delta P}$ below the
normal hydropenic value of 35 mm Hg are predicted to increase the frac-
tional clearance of M. However, increases in $\overline{\Delta P}$ above this value will
have little effect because as $\overline{\Delta P}$ rises, both the convective and diffusive
components of macromolecular transport will increase in proportion to
the increase in GFR. Thus, increases in Q_A and $\overline{\Delta P}$, both expected to increase the filtration rate of water, are predicted to have different effects
on the fractional clearance of macromolecular solutes.

Figure 2C reveals that increases in the value of C_A are predicted to
act like decreases in the value of $\overline{\Delta P}$, as both of the maneuvers alter the
mean net ultrafiltration pressure, $\overline{P}_{UF}$, in the same direction. Thus, in-

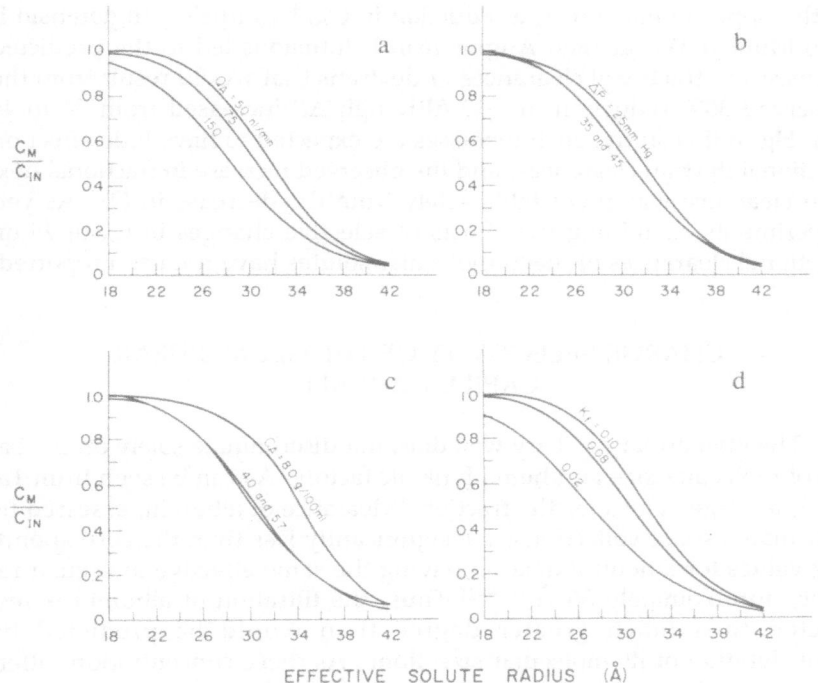

EFFECTIVE SOLUTE RADIUS (Å)

Figure 2. The theoretical relationships among fractional clearance (C_M/C_{IN}) of a neutral macromolecule (M), effective radius of M, and selective variations in the initial glomerular capillary plasma flow rate (Q_A) (A), the mean transcapillary hydraulic pressure difference ($\overline{\Delta P}$) (B), the initial glomerular capillary plasma protein concentration (C_A) (C), and the ultrafiltration coefficient (K_f) (D). Input quantities representative of the normal hydropenic Munich–Wistar rat were $Q_A = 75$ nl/min, $\overline{\Delta P} = 36$ mm Hg, $C_A = 5.7$ g/dl, $K_f = 0.08$ nl/s per mm Hg, and pore radius $= 50$ Å. (Reprinted with permission from Brenner et al.[17])

creases in C_A above the usual hydropenic value of 5.7 g/dl should increase fractional clearance, whereas decreases in C_A should exert little effect. Finally, variations in the value of K_f from the normal of 0.08 nl/s per mm Hg will produce directionally similar changes in the fractional clearance of M (Fig. 2D).

These theoretical predictions have been tested in a study by Chang and associates[3] in which fractional clearances of neutral dextrans were determined in Munich–Wistar rats at normal hydropenic values of Q_A and at elevated flows induced by plasma-volume expansion. When Q_A was raised from 70 nl/min to 220 nl/min, the fractional dextran clearances were reduced to levels very similar to those predicted by theoretical considerations. Subsequently, Bohrer and co-workers[18] studied the effects of the opposite maneuver, a reduction in Q_A, by infusing angiotensin II into Munich–Wistar rats. Angiotensin II infusions led to the predicted increases in fractional clearances of dextrans that would result from the observed 30% reduction in Q_A. Although $\overline{\Delta P}$ increased from 34 to 44 mm Hg in this study, such increases are expected to have little effect on fractional dextran clearances, and the observed increase in fractional dextran clearance was predictable solely from the decrease in Q_A. As yet, experiments examining the effects of selective changes in C_A or K_f on fractional clearances of macromolecular solutes have not been reported.

CHARGE SELECTIVITY OF THE GLOMERULAR CAPILLARY WALL

The glomerular capillary wall does not discriminate solely on the basis of molecular size and hemodynamic factors. As can be seen from Table I, average values for the fractional clearance of albumin, assessed by Bowman's space collections, are significantly less than the corresponding values for a neutral dextran having the same effective molecular radius, approximately 36 Å.[3,19-21] Thus, the filtration of albumin is restricted to a much greater degree than would be predicted by consideration of its molecular size alone. As these concentration differences already exist in Bowman's space,[3,19-21] they are not caused by protein reabsorption by the renal tubules. Considerable evidence is now available that this relative restriction of albumin filtration results from the fact that albumin is a polyanion at physiological pH and that the glomerulus possesses a charge-selective barrier to macromolecular filtration.

Chang and co-workers[2] examined the role of molecular charge by studying the sieving characteristics of dextran sulfate, an anionic derivative of dextran. Figure 1 compares the results for dextran and dextran sulfate (solid circles, left and middle panels). Neutral dextrans are not measurably restricted until effective radii exceed 20 Å, whereas dextran sulfates exhibit restricted filtration over the entire range of molecular radii studied. As with neutral dextrans, fractional clearances of anionic dextrans decrease progressively with increasing molecular radius, but additionally, for each radius studied, the fractional clearance of dextran sulfate is less than the corresponding clearance of a neutral dextran of equivalent size. At very large values of effective molecular radius, the differences between these two dextran species lessen, as the fractional clearances of both forms approach zero. As neither dextran nor dextran sulfate is significantly secreted or reabsorbed by the renal tubules, these

Table I. Fractional Clearance of Albumin Compared with That of Neutral Dextran, Dextran Sulfate, and Diethylaminoethyl (DEAE) Dextran of Similar Molecular Size in the Normal Munich–Wistar Rat[a]

Macromolecule	Molecular radius (Å)	$C_M C_{IN}$
Albumin[21]	36	0.01[b]
Neutral dextran[2,3]	36	0.15 ± 0.02
Dextran sulfate[2]	36	0.01 ± 0.002
DEAE dextran[1]	36	0.42 ± 0.06

[a]Values are means ± S.E.M. Adapted from Brenner et al.,[17] with permission.
[b]Bowman's space/plasma water ratio of albumin.

studies suggest that molecular charge is another important determinant of macromolecular filtration rate. Table I indicates that the fractional clearance of dextran sulfate with a molecular radius of 36 Å approaches the fractional clearance of similarly sized albumin. The greater restriction to the filtration of circulating polyanions such as albumin and dextran sulfate most likely results from the presence of some fixed, negatively charged component or components of the glomerular capillary wall. This same conclusion was also reached by Rennke, Cotran, and Venkatachalam.[22]

As electrostatic interactions at the glomerular capillary wall retard the filtration of polyanions, they might enhance the filtration of circulating polycations. Rennke and co-workers[22-24] have provided support for this hypothesis in experiments using cationic forms of ferritin and horseradish peroxidase. These polycations were transported across glomerular capillary walls to a much greater extent than were their corresponding neutral species. Similarly, Fig. 1 (right panel, solid circles) compares the fractional clearances of a cationic form of dextran, diethylaminoethyl (DEAE) dextran to neutral dextran (left panel, solid circles). These results, obtained by Bohrer and associates,[1] revealed that the fractional clearances of cationic dextrans are greatly enhanced relative to neutral dextrans at molecular radii of sufficient size so that significant restriction to the filtration of neutral molecules exists. As shown in Table I, DEAE dextrans with a molecular radius of 36 Å have a fractional clearance of approximately 0.4, a value much in excess of the corresponding clearances of similarly sized neutral dextrans, dextran sulfates, and albumin. This "facilitated" filtration of cationic species provides further support for the existence of significant electrostatic interactions between circulating charged macromolecules and negatively charged components in the glomerular capillary wall.

Morphological studies using cationic "stains" such as colloidal iron,

alcian blue, ruthenium red, and lysosyme have demonstrated fixed negative charges in all layers of the normal glomerular capillary wall.[25-31]
These substances bind to a number of structures including the surfaces
of endothelial and epithelial cells and the glomerular basement membrane. Kanwar and co-workers[32-36] have suggested several biochemical
components of these structures that may act as anionic sites, including
the sialyl groups of heteropolysaccharides, the carboxyl groups of collagenous or noncollagenous glycopeptides, and the sulfate groups of
glycosaminoglycans.

Recently, Deen and associates[37] developed a theoretical model to account for the charge selectivity of the glomerular capillary wall. This
model incorporates terms for the size-selective and hemodynamic properties of the glomerular sieve, discussed above, but additionally assumes
that the capillary wall has a homogeneous distribution of fixed negative
charges and that Donnan equilibria exist at the surfaces of this membrane. By applying this mathematical construct to the dextran sieving
data discussed above, Deen and co-workers[37] estimated that the
glomerular capillary wall of the rat has an apparent fixed negative charge
concentration of 120–170 mEq/liter. A more detailed mathematical discussion of these calculations is beyond the scope of this review, and the
reader is referred to the original article of Deen, Satvat, and Jamieson.[37]

EFFECTS OF MOLECULAR CONFIGURATION
ON THE FILTRATION OF MACROMOLECULES

The theories of size and charge selectivity of the glomerular capillary
wall, discussed above, are in part based on comparisons of the filtration
rates of macromolecules of very different structures (dextran polymers
and globular proteins). In addition to differences in charge, it has been
suggested that the shapes or configurations of these molecules might also
influence their fractional clearance.[38-40] Two studies have specifically examined this question and have demonstrated that molecular configuration does affect macromolecular filtration across the glomerular capillary
wall. Bohrer et al.[40] compared the fractional clearance of neutral dextran,
a flexible coil in solution, with ficoll, a rigid, cross-linked polymer, in
Munich–Wistar rats. At any effective molecular radius, the flexible dextran was more readily filtered than the rigid, spherical ficoll. At the molecular radius of albumin (36 Å), the average fractional clearance of ficoll
was about one-half that of dextran. As the magnitude of this effect was
relatively small, this study suggested that even if albumin acts as a rigid
sphere similar to ficoll, molecular configuration only accounts for a mi-

nor part of the large difference in the relative clearances of neutral dextrans and albumin. Accordingly, molecular configuration seemed to exert relatively little influence on the transglomerular passage of macromolecules as compared with molecular charge.

Somewhat different results have been reported by Rennke and Venkatachalam[38] who examined this same issue by comparing the simultaneous fractional clearances of native horseradish peroxidase (a protein of molecular radius of 28 Å) and a neutral dextran of similar dimensions. The mean fractional clearance of the protein was approximately one-seventh that of dextran, suggesting that conformational differences between globular molecules (proteins) and random coil molecules (dextrans) played a more significant role in the control of macromolecular sieving.

In summary, the normal glomerular capillary wall acts as a barrier to the filtration of plasma proteins and other macromolecules while at the same time permitting a high rate of fluid filtration. Experiments using a variety of charged and neutral tracers have established that this selectivity is based on the ability of the glomerulus to act as both a size-selective and a charge-selective filter. These same techniques, applied to patients and animals with diseases of the renal glomerulus, reveal that significant proteinuria results when alterations in the structure of the glomerular capillary wall change its size- and/or charge-selective properties.

LOCATION OF THE FILTRATION BARRIER
TO MACROMOLECULES

Ultrastructural tracer studies[41] indicate that macromolecules traverse the glomerular capillary wall via an extracellular route. This pathway includes, in sequence, the endothelial fenestrae, the glomerular basement membrane (GBM), and the filtration slit diaphragms. Using native horse-spleen ferritin (effective radius ~61 Å) as a tracer substance, Farquhar, Wissig, and Palade[42] concluded that the GBM was the main barrier to filtration of this protein. However, Graham and Karnovsky[41] subsequently demonstrated that human myeloperoxidase, with an effective radius roughly two-thirds that of ferritin, traversed the GBM and was hindered in the region of the filtration slit disphragm. Accordingly, these authors suggested that the slit diaphragm was the main barrier to circulating macromolecules. Venkatachalam and co-workers[43] studied the filtration characteristics of still another enzymatic tracer, catalase. Their experiments produced evidence that restriction to protein filtration occurred both at the level of the GBM and at the slit diaphragms. These authors subsequently advanced the "double-barrier hypothesis," which proposed that the GBM functioned as a coarse filter, whereas the filtration slit diaphragms served as a finer screen. However, even this compromise failed to resolve the issue, and Caulfield and Farquhar[44] later obtained further evidence that the GBM was the sole site of the filtration barrier in their studies using neutral dextrans as tracers.

It is important to recognize that these morphological studies were interpreted at a time prior to the realization that the glomerular capillary wall was capable of charge as well as size discrimination. Therefore, it is interesting to examine whether electrostatic factors may have influenced the conclusions derived from the various ultrastructural studies cited above. Native ferritins and catalase are anionic molecules, and studies using these tracers[42,43] suggested that the GBM was the main barrier. A similar conclusion was reached when neutral dextrans were employed.[44] However, when cationic tracers such as myeloperoxidase[41] were studied, the evidence pointed toward a more distal barrier located at the filtration slit diaphragms. Apparently, the major glomerular capillary barrier to the filtration of macromolecules varies with the charge of the test substance.

Morphological studies using cationic "stains" such as colloidal iron, alcian blue, ruthenium red, and lysozyme have demonstrated fixed negative charges in all layers of the normal glomerular capillary wall.[25-36] These substances bind to a number of structures, including the surfaces of endothelial and epithelial cells and the GBM. Kanwar and associates[32-36] have suggested that the sialyl groups of heteropolysaccharides, the carboxyl groups of collagenous or noncollagenous glycopeptides, and the sulfate groups of glycosaminoglycans all contribute to the fixed negative charge properties of the glomerular capillary wall. Cytochemical staining[33] and chemical analyses[34] have demonstrated that the glycosaminoglycan heparin sulfate is a major anionic component of the GBM. Furthermore, treatment of kidneys with heparinase, an enzyme that removes most heparin sulfate, leads to increased glomerular permeability to anionic native ferritin molecules.[35] It seems, therefore, that the GBM plays an important role in the charge-selective properties of the glomerular capillary wall.

Recent studies suggest that firm attachment of the epithelial foot processes to the GBM is also necessary for normal barrier function. Kanwar and Rosenzweig[36] reported that detachment of the visceral epithelium from the GBM, induced by either perfusing kidneys with neuraminidase or administering puromycin aminonucleoside, led to increased glomerular permeability to anionic ferritin, mainly in areas of the capillary wall where the epithelium was detached. Furthermore, increased permeability occurred even though the GBM at these sites appeared structurally intact.

Taken together, these morphological studies of glomerular permeability suggest that all layers of the glomerular capillary wall contribute to normal barrier function. However, Ryan and Karnovsky[45] have suggested that the glomerular localization of some macromolecular tracers may be influenced by cessation of blood flow and tissue fixation, conditions that existed in most of the experiments discussed above. In addition, purely theoretical considerations predict that the glomerular filtration barrier must be located close to the blood–capillary wall interface, i.e., at the endothelial cell.[46] If not, then large molecules driven by transcapillary convective and diffusive gradients would be expected to accumulate within the capillary wall. Eventually, these molecules would clog the filter and impair its efficiency. This hypothesis is supported by studies that indicate that the glomerular endothelial cells are richly endowed with fixed negative charges.[47] Furthermore, Rennke et al.[24] have demonstrated that although some anionic ferritin molecules penetrate to the GBM, significant restriction occurs at the level of the endothelium. Similar macromolecule–endothelial interactions have also been demonstrated in nonrenal vascular tissues.[47]

In summary, despite extensive study, the exact anatomic location of the barrier to the transglomerular passage of macromolecules remains uncertain. It is likely that circulating polyanions are significanctly hindered by the negatively charged endothelium. For neutral macromolecules, the GBM is generally considered to provide the major restrictive influence. For more cationic substances, most evidence suggests that the epithelial filtration slit diaphragms exert significant barrier function.

REFERENCES

1. Bohrer MP, Baylis C, Humes HD, et al: Permselectivity of the glomerular capillary wall: Facilitated filtration of circulation polycations. *J Clin Invest* 61:72–78, 1978
2. Chang RLS, Deen WM, Robertson CR, et al: Permselectivity of the glomerular capillary wall. III. Restricted transport of polyanions. *Kidney Int* 8:212–218, 1975
3. Chang RLS, Ueki IF, Troy JL, et al: Permselectivity of the glomerular capillary wall to macromolecules. II. Experimental studies in rats using neutral dextran. *Biophys J* 15:887–906, 1975
4. Arturson G, Groth T, Grotte G: Human glomerular membrane porosity and filtration pressure: Dextran clearance data analyzed by theoretical models. *Clin Sci* 40:137–158, 1971
5. Gassée MP: Effect of acetylcholine on glomerular sieving of macromolecules. *Pfluegers Arch* 342:239–254, 1973

6. Gassée JP, Dubois R, Staroukine M, et al: Determination of glomerular intracapillary and transcapillary pressure gradients from sieving data. III. The effects of angiotensin II. *Pfluegers Arch* 367:15–24, 1976
7. Hardwicke J. Cameron JS, Harrison JF, et al: Proteinuria studied by clearances of individual macromolecules, in Manuel Y, Revillard JP, Betuel H (eds): *Proteins in Normal and Pathological Urine*. Baltimore, University Park Press, 1970, pp 111–152
8. Jamison RL: Intrarenal heterogeneity. The case for two functionally dissimilar populations of nephrons in the mammalian kidney. *Am J Med* 54:281–289, 1973
9. Lambert PP, Dubois R, Decoodt P, et al: Determination of glomerular intracapillary and transcapillary pressure gradients from sieving data. II. A physiological study in the normal dog. *Pfluegers Arch* 359:1–22, 1975
10. Verniory M, Dubois R, Decoodt P, et al: Measurement of the permeability of biological membranes: Application to the glomerular wall. *J Gen Physiol* 62:489–507, 1973
11. Pappenheimer JR: Passage of molecules through capillary walls. *Physiol Rev* 33:387–423, 1953
12. Pappenheimer JR, Renkin EM, Borrero LM: Filtration diffusion and molecular sieving through peripheral capillary membranes. A contribution to the pore theory of capillary permeability. *Am J Physiol* 167:13–46, 1951
13. Renkin EM, Gilmore JP: Glomerular filtration, in Orloff J, Berliner RW (eds): *Handbook of Physiology, Section 8: Renal Physiology*. Washington, American Physiological Society, 1973, pp 185–248
14. Deen WM, Bohrer MP, Brenner BM: Macromolecule transport across glomerular capillaries: Application of pore theory. *Kidney Int* 16:353–365, 1979
15. Deen WM, Satvat B: Determinants of the glomerular filtration of proteins. *Am J Physiol* 241:F162–F170, 1981
16. Chang RLS, Robertson CR, Deen WM, et al: Permselectivity of the glomerular capillary wall to macromolecules. I. Theoretical considerations. *Biophys J* 15:861–886, 1975
17. Brenner BM, Bohrer MP, Baylis C, et al: Determinants of glomerular permselectivity: Insights derived from observations in vivo. *Kidney Int* 12:229–237, 1977
18. Bohrer MP, Troy JL, Deen WM, et al: Mechanism of angiotensin II-induced proteinuria in the rat. *Am J Physiol* 233:F13–F21, 1977
19. Brenner BM, Troy JL, Daugherty TM: The dynamics of glomerular ultrafiltration in the rat. *J Clin Invest* 50:1776–1780, 1971
20. Eisenbach GM, van Liew JB, Manz N, et al: Effect of angiotensin on the filtration of protein in the rat kidney: A micropuncture study. *Kidney Int* 8:80–87, 1975
21. Gaizutis M, Pesce AJ, Lewy JE: Determination of nanogram amounts of albumin by radioimmunoassay. *Microchem J* 17:327–337, 1972
22. Rennke HG, Cotran RS, Venkatachalam MA: Role of molecular charge in glomerular permeability: Tracer studies with cationized ferritins. *J Cell Biol* 67:638–646, 1975
23. Rennke HG, Patel Y, Venkatachalam MA: Effect of molecular charge on glomerular permeability to proteins in the rat: Clearance studies using neutral, anionic and cationic horseradish peroxidase. *Kidney Int* 13:278–288, 1978
24. Rennke HG, Venkatachalam MA: Glomerular permeability: In vivo tracer studies with polyanionic and polycationic ferritins. *Kidney Int* 11:44–53, 1977
25. Blau EB, Haas DE: Glomerular sialic acid and proteinuria in human renal disease. *Lab Invest* 28:477–481, 1973
26. Caulfield JP, Farquhar MG: Distribution of anionic sites in normal and nephrotic glomerular basement membranes. *J Cell Biol* 70:92a, 1976
27. Jones DB: Mucosubstances of the glomerulus. *Lab Invest* 21:119–125, 1969

28. Latta H, Johnston, WH, Stanley TM: Sialoglycoproteins and filtration barriers in the glomerular capillary wall. *J Ultrastruct Res* 51:354–376, 1975
29. Michael AF, Blau E, Vernier RL: Glomerular polyanion alteration in aminonucleoside nephrosis. *Lab Invest* 23:649–657, 1970
30. Seiler MW, Rennke HG, Cotran RS, et al: Pathogenesis of polycation-induced alterations ("fusion") of glomerular epithelium. *Lab Invest* 36:48, 1977
31. Seiler MW, Venkatachalam MA, Cotran RS: Glomerular epithelium: Structural alterations induced by polycations. *Science* 189:390–393, 1975
32. Kanwar YS, Farquhar MG: Anionic sites in the glomerular basement membrane. In vivo and in vitro localization to the luminae by cationic probes. *J Cell Biol* 81:137–153, 1979
33. Kanwar YS, Farquhar MG: Presence of heparin sulfate in the glomerular basement membrane. *Proc Natl Acad Sci USA* 76:1303–1307, 1979
34. Kanwar YS, Farquhar MG: Isolation of glycosaminoglycans (heparin sulfate) from glomerular basement membranes. *Proc Natl Acad Sci USA* 76:4493–4497, 1979
35. Kanwar YS, Linker A, Farquhar MG: Increased permeability of the glomerular basement membrane to ferritin after removal of glycosaminoglycans (heparin sulfate) by enzyme digestion. *J Cell Biol* 86:688–693, 1980
36. Kanwar YS, Rosenzweig LJ: Altered glomerular permeability as a result of focal detachment of the visceral epithelium. *Kidney Int* 21:565–574, 1982
37. Deen WM, Satvat B, Jamieson JM: Theoretical model of glomerular filtration of charged solutes. *Am J Physiol* 238:F126–F139, 1980
38. Rennke HG, Venkatachalam MA: Glomerular permeability of macromolecules: Effect of molecular configuration on the fractional clearance of uncharged dextran and neutral horseradish peroxidase in the rat. *J Clin Invest* 63:713–717, 1979
39. Rennke HG, Venkatachalam MA: Structural determinants of glomerular permselectivity. *Fed Proc* 36:2619–2626, 1977
40. Bohrer MP, Deen WM, Robertson CR, et al: Influence of molecular configuration on the passage of macromolecules across the glomerular capillary wall. *J Gen Physiol* 74:583–593, 1979
41. Graham RC, Karnovsky MJ: Glomerular permeability. Ultrastructural cytochemical studies using peroxidases as protein tracers. *J Exp Med* 124:1123–1124, 1966
42. Farquhar JG, Wissig SL, Palade GE: Glomerular permeability. I. Ferritin transfer across the normal glomerular capillary wall. *J Exp Med* 113:47–66, 1961
43. Venkatachalam MA, Karnovsky MJ, Fahimi HD, et al: An ultrastructural study of glomerular permeability using catalase and peroxidase as tracer proteins. *J Exp Med* 132:1153–1167, 1970
44. Caulfield JP, Farquhar MG: The permeability of glomerular capillaries to graded dextrans. *J Cell Biol* 63:883–903, 1974
45. Ryan GB, Karnovsky MJ: Distribution of endogenous albumin in the rat glomerulus: Role of hemodynamic factors in glomerular barrier function. *Kidney Int* 9:36–45, 1976
46. Lassen N: Large molecules, in Crone CC, Lassen NA (eds): *Capillary Permeability*. New York, Academic Press, 1970, pp 549–551
47. Simionescu N, Simionescu M, Palade GF: Differentiated microdomains on the luminal surface of the capillary endothelium. 1. Preferential distribution of anionic sites. *J Cell Biol* 90:605–613, 1981
48. Brenner BM, Hostetter TH, Humes HD: Molecular basis of proteinuria of glomerular origin. *N Engl J Med* 298:826, 1978

2

In Vivo Evaluation of Glomerular Permselectivity in Normal and Nephrotic Man

BRYAN D. MYERS

PERMEABILITY PROPERTIES OF THE GLOMERULAR FILTER

Glomerular filtration is the first step in the process of urine formation. The rate at which ultrafiltrate is formed is governed by the Starling forces. In order to achieve the rapid rate of filtration required to regulate the composition and volume of the body fluids, glomerular capillaries possess unique functional and structural characteristics. A striking example is an extraordinarily high hydraulic permeability. In comparison to capillaries from various other microvascular beds, it has been shown that glomerular capillaries are one to two orders of magnitude more permeable to water than are other capillaries.[1]

Despite this extraordinary permeability to water (and small solutes), the glomerular capillary wall imposes an extremely efficient barrier to the passage of plasma proteins.[2] This permselectivity can be recognized by examining the extent to which the glomerular capillary wall discriminates among molecules of varying size. Unlike small modecules the size of inulin or below, which permeate the capillary wall as freely as water, the transport of substances of increasingly greater size diminishes progressively, normally reaching very low values as the size of serum albumin is approached. For this reason, all but the smallest plasma proteins are normally restricted from passage into Bowman's space.

The most rigorous demonstration of this permselectivity comes from the finding that fluid sampled from Bowman's space conforms very closely to that of an ideal ultrafiltrate of plasma.[3] In the rat, such meas-

BRYAN D. MYERS • Department of Medicine, Division of Nephrology, Stanford University School of Medicine, Stanford, California 94305.

urements clearly indicate that inulin and substances smaller than inulin appear in glomerular filtrate in essentially the same concentration as in plasma water, whereas serum albumin is filtered to a much lesser extent.[4,5] The application of ultramicroscopic disk electrophoresis to nanoliter samples of glomerular ultrafiltrate or proximal tubule fluid obtained by micropuncture techniques indicates that albumin concentration in glomerular ultrafiltrate approximates 1 mg/dl. In contrast, plasma albumin concentration ranges between 3 and 4 g/dl. The Bowman's space fluid-to-plasma albumin concentration ratio (a quantity known as a sieving coefficient) therefore is less than 0.1% of that of inulin.

PERMSELECTIVITY OF THE NORMAL GLOMERULAR CAPILLARY WALL

The mechanisms whereby the normal glomerular capillary wall (GCW) restricts the transmural passage of large plasma proteins while offering little resistance to the filtration of water and small solutes have been explored extensively in recent years. The effects of the molecular properties of several proteins on glomerular selectivity are summarized in Table I. In these examples, either direct sampling by the micropuncture technique[4,5] or precise determination of fractional protein reabsorption[6] has been used to determine the Bowman's space-to-plasma concentration ratio for various proteins in the rat. This ratio is known as the *sieving coefficient* (Θ) of the GCW for a given protein. Transmural transport of the largest proteins (albumin and γ-globulin) is considerably more restricted than that of the smallest proteins (monomeric immunoglublin light chains). A clear trend towards progressive restriction of transmural transport with increasing size of the test protein only becomes obvious, however, when the molecular charge of each protein is taken into account. Thus, the inverse relationship between the sieving coefficient and Stokes radius of either anionic (isoelectric point <7.4) or cationic (isoelectric point >7.4) proteins indicates that the glomerular capillary wall has the properties of a size-selective filter. On the other hand, the greater restriction of anionic than cationic proteins of equivalent or similar radius points to the existence within the glomerular capillary wall of an electrostatic barrier (or charge-selective filter).[2]

Because of the inaccessibility of Bowman's space and the technical limitations of measuring accurately protein concentration in nanoliter samples of Bowman's space fluid, the number of observations of the type shown in Table I is limited. Glomerular permselectivity has, however, been extensively studied with the use of the fractional clearance tech-

Table I. Sieving Coefficients for Various Proteins

		MW	Stokes radius (Å)	Isoelectric point	BS/P concentration ratio (θ)
Immunoglobulin	(a)	22,000	24	8.9	0.495
light chains	(b)	22,000	24	4.8	0.021
Horseradish	(a)	40,000	31	9.5–10.5	0.276
peroxidase[a]	(b)	40,000	29	3.7	0.007
Albumin		69,000	36	4.9	0.001
γ-Globulin		180,000	55	6.6–10	0.003

[a]The Bowman's space concentration of HRP in this example has actually been derived from knowledge of precise values of the fractional clearance and fractional reabsorption.

nique.[2] The fractional clearance of a test macromolecule (M) is defined as the clearance of M divided by the glomerular filtration rate of water (GFR). With the clearance of inulin used to measure the GFR, fractional clearance is calculated from the urine (U) and plasma (P) concentration of M and inulin (IN) as follows:

$$\text{Fractional clearance of } M = (U/P)_M/(U/P)_{IN} \qquad (1)$$

If, like inulin, the test macromolecule is neither reabsorbed nor secreted by the tubule, the fractional clearance of M will be exactly equal to the Bowman's space-to-plasma concentration ratio of M, the sieving coefficient (θ). Thus, for a test macromolecule with these special properties,

$$\theta = (U/P)_M/(U/P)_{IN} \qquad (2)$$

and only urine and plasma samples are required to calculate θ.

Size Selectivity

Because proteins normally undergo tubular reabsorption, they are unsuitable as test macromolecules when fractional clearances are used to probe the glomerular filtration barrier. However, two nonprotein polymers, dextran and polyvinylpyrrolidone (PVP), are neither reabsorbed nor secreted by the tubule and have been extensively used for this purpose.[7] The size-selective properties of the GCW have been demonstrated by using uncharged polydisperse preparations of these polymers. The absence of charge eliminates the consequences of electrical interaction between the permeating macromolecule and charged components of the GCW: polydispersion with respect to molecular size permits the determination of fractional clearance over a range of molecular sizes.

An example of this approach is illustrated in Fig. 1. Here, an uncharged preparation of dextran, a polymer of D—glucopyranose, has been infused into 20 healthy volunteers to characterize the molecular sieving properties of the normal human GCW. Dextran fractional clearances (or sieving coefficients, Θ) are plotted as a function of effective dextran radius, with the latter determined by its elution from calibrated gel-chromatographic columns. A value of 1.0 on the ordinate represents equality of dextran and inulin clearances and indicates no measurable restriction to transport of dextran across the GCW when effective molecular radius is 20 Å or less. With increasing size, however, dextrans are progressively restricted, as judged by a rapidly declining value for Θ. As shown in Fig. 1, fractional clearances approach zero, indicating dextran impermeance, when dextran radius exceeds 60 Å. It is noteworthy that strikingly similar fractional clearance profiles to that shown for man in Fig. 1 have been reported for neutral dextrans and PVP in other mammalian species, including the rat,[7] dog,[8] and rabbit.[9]

The most useful theoretical descriptions of macromolecule transport across the glomerular capillary wall are based on the concept of hindered movement of solutes through water-filled pores.[10] By such theoretical analyses, the dextran filtration data in Fig. 1 are accurately predicted by models that envision transport as taking place through numerous identical cylindrical pores with a radius of 55 Å.[11] Application of dextran or PVP filtration data from the rat, dog, and rabbit to the same isoporous theory reveals similar values for pore radius in these species.

For a more complete discussion of the theories of partitioning and hindered particle motion in the context of glomerular filtration and for a detailed description of the pore model of solute transport, the reader is referred to a recent review by Deen et al.[12]

Charge-Selective Barrier

The large disparity between the Bowman's space-to-plasma water concentration ratio of albumin ($\Theta = 0.001$, Table I) and that derived for a dextran of equivalent gel chromatographic radius ($\Theta = 0.25$, Fig. 1) points strongly to an influence of molecular charge on the transglomerular transport of circulating macromolecules. As stated previously, albumin behaves as a polyanion in physiological solution. Conversely, the various subclasses of IgG are predominantly neutral or cationic. It is interesting to note, therefore, that Θ for IgG in the rat is quite similar to that derived for a dextran of equivalent radius, 55 Å, in man (0.003 vs. 0.01).

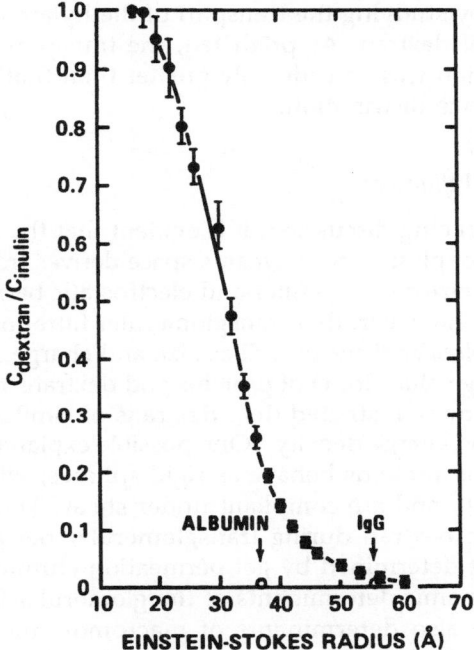

Figure 1. The fractional dextran clearance profile of the normal glomerular capillary wall as determined in 20 healthy adult volunteers. Fractional dextran clearances are plotted as a function of the Stokes radius of the dextran. The vertical bars represent one standard error of the mean. The Bowman's space-to-plasma concentration ratio for albumin and IgG in the rat (O) are shown for comparison.

To test the effects of molecular charge, Bohrer et al. used the fractional clearance technique to study transglomerular transport in the rat.[13] They compared uncharged dextrans to dextran sulfate, an anionic polymer similar in structure to neutral dextran. In keeping with the findings for various proteins in Table I, anionic dextran sulfate transport was restricted relative to that of neutral dextrans over the entire range of molecular sizes examined. Moreover, the fractional clearance (Θ) of dextran sulfate of radius 36 Å, averaged 0.001, a value considerably less than that for neutral dextrans of the same size and more closely approaching the value of Θ observed for albumin. This observed restriction of the filtration of polyanions relative to neutral macromolecules is inferred to be the result of electrostatic retardation by fixed, negatively charged components of the glomerular capillary wall (vide infra).[14] That electrical interaction between the negatively charged glomerular capillary wall and circulating macromolecules is an important feature of the filtration barrier was then confirmed by studying the transport of diethylaminoethyldextran, a cationic form of dextran. As predicted, the transport of this cationic dextran preparation was considerably greater than that of neutral dextrans of similar size distribution.

Other Biophysical Influences

From the foregoing discussion, it is evident that the formation of an ideal ultrafiltrate of plasma in Bowman's space derives from the behavior of the GCW as a size-selective filter and electrostatic barrier. It is important to point out, however, that transglomerular filtration appears to be influenced by *molecular shape* as well as size and charge. Comparison of the corresponding values for Θ of proteins and dextrans reveals that proteins are always more restricted than dextrans of similar gel chromatographic radius and charge density.[6] One possible explanation for the disparity may be that proteins behave as rigid spheres, whereas dextrans display asphericity and are compliant under shear. Thus, the effective radius of a given dextran during transglomerular permeation may be smaller than that determined by gel permeation chromatography.

The hemodynamic determinants of the glomerular filtration rate of water (GFR) are also determinants of macromolecule filtration.[12] In general, hemodynamic changes that result in a low filtration fraction (GFR/renal plasma flow) will reduce Θ for a given macromolecule, whereas those that elevate the filtration fraction will have an opposite effect. This is because mean intraluminal concentration of a relatively impermeant macromolecule will increase with distance along the glomerular capillaries in parallel with the fraction of plasma water that is removed from the capillary by filtration. Both diffusive transport (down the plasma to Bowman's space concentration gradient) and convective transport (bulk flow) will be increased at high versus low plasma macromolecule concentration and will thus change in parallel with the filtration fraction.

STRUCTURAL CORRELATES OF THE FILTRATION BARRIER

The wall of the mammalian glomerular capillary is a complex structure comprising three distinct layers (Fig. 2). These are (1) an inner layer of fenestrated cytoplasm of endothelial origin, (2) a middle layer formed by the glomerular basement membrane (GBM), a laminated structure composed of types IV and V collagen, and (3) an outer layer of interdigitating cytoplasmic processes of epithelial origin known as foot

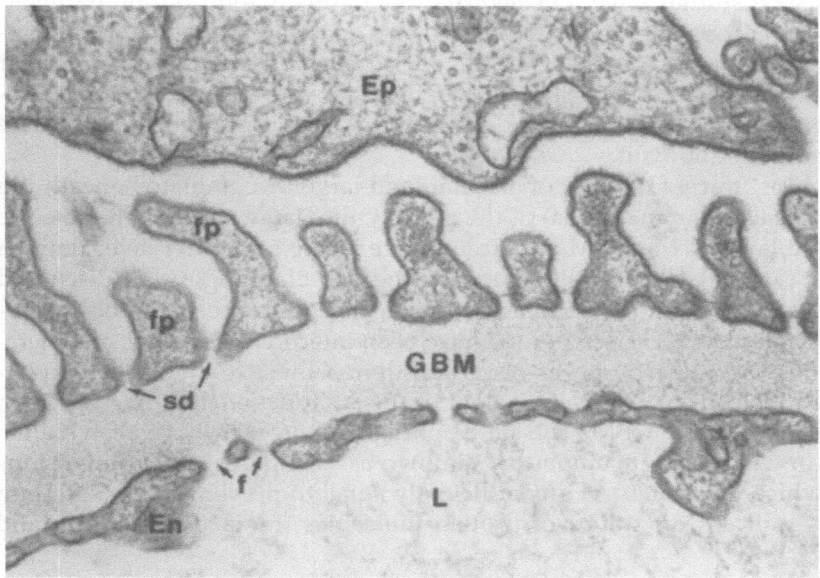

Figure 2. Ultrastructure of the glomerular capillary wall: The inner layer is composed of endothelial cytoplasm (En), which is fenestrated (f). The middle layer is the glomerular basement membrane (GBM), which has a dense central lamina and rare inner and outer laminae. The outer layer is composed of epithelial cell (Ep) foot processes (fp). These areanchored in the GBM and separated by filtration slits sealed off below by a slit diaphragm (sd).

processes. Because of the large width of the endothelial fenestrae and of the epithelial filtration slits (the spaces that separate adjacent foot processes), approximately 1000 Å and 300 Å, respectively, neither the inner endothelial nor outer epithelial layers of the GCW would appear at first sight capable of serving as major barriers for the transmural passage of plasma proteins. On the basis of its continous or uninterrupted nature, the GBM, by contrast, was considered for many years to be the primary barrier to protein filtration.

In recent years, a more detailed structural characterization of the filtration barrier has emerged. This has resulted, in large part, from a morphological technique in which large tracer molecules are used. In these experiments, a soluble, particulate, and electron-dense tracer (usually a large protein such as ferritin or a polymer of similar size) is injected into the cirulation of an experimental animal. The distribution of the electron-dense tracer particles within the GCW is then localized by high-resolution electron microscopy.[15]

Such studies have revealed that the pathway followed by permeating tracer macromolecules into Bowman's space is extracellular. It is composed (in sequential order) of the endothelial fenestrae, the glomerular basement membrane, a slit diaphragm that spans the space between adjacent epithelial processes, and the latter space itself, which is referred to as a filtration slit.

Most tracers the size of albumin and larger accumulate beneath the dense layer (lamina densa) of the GBM. Other large tracers penetrate the dense layer of the GBM and accumulate in the rare outer layer (lamina rara externa) of the GBM beneath the slit diaphragm. As discussed above, the results of studies in which the clearance of probe macromolecules has been determined have been interpreted in terms of a membrane perforated by pores of certain dimensions. It should be emphasized that no structural equivalent of these "functional" pores has been visualized in the GBM. The slit diaphragms, however, have been shown to contain rectangular apertures known as "slit pores," the dimensions of which (50 × 120 Å) are sufficiently small to prevent the penetration of significant quantities of protein molecules the size of albumin and larger.[16]

The technique of particulate tracer localization has also provided insights into the nature of the electrostatic filtration barrier. In keeping with the differential clearance of test macromolecules of varying charge, the molecular charge of a given tracer molecule has been shown to influence the facility with which it penetrates the GCW. Thus, for example, ferritin (radius = 61 Å) in its native anionic form has been shown to accumulate at the level of endothelial fenestrae and in the lamina rara interna of the GBM. Cationized forms of ferritin, by contrast, penetrate the dense layer of the GBM and accumulate beneath the slit diaphragm.[17] With the use of cytochemical techniques, it has been shown that all three layers of the GCW are richly endowed with negatively charged components. The anionic components of the GBM are glycosamine glycans, which are densely distributed throughout the rare and dense layers of this structure.[18] The coating of the cell membrane surrounding endothelial cells and epithelial foot processes, in contrast, is composed largely of anionic glycoproteins that are rich in sialic acid residues.[19]

The relationship between the functional concept of a "porous" membrane and the ultrastructure of the GCW is most easily understood when the latter is envisioned as a single unit. In other words, the respective anionic glycoprotein coats of endothelial cells and epithelial foot processes may be thought of as occupying the endothelial fenestrae and epithelial filtration slits. These coats (referred to as glycocalyces) and the adjacent glycosamine-glycan-rich basement membrane may be regarded as a continuous anionic polymeric matrix extending from the capillary lumen to Bowman's space. The hydrated "pores" in the interior of this matrix are effectively narrowed for polyanions (electrostatic retardation) and widened for polycations (electrical enhancement). When the permeating molecule is sufficiently large, however, it will be excluded by the pores within the matrix on the basis of its size alone and irrespective of its molecular charge.[15]

EVALUATION OF THE HUMAN FILTRATION BARRIER IN NEPHROTIC PATIENTS

Differential Protein Clearances

A variety of primary glomerular diseases are associated with increased glomerular permeability to large plasma proteins. When urinary protein excretion reaches nephrotic proportions (>3.5 g/24 h), the urinary concentration of even very large plasma proteins such as α_2-macroglobulin (MW 720,000) may reach easily measurable levels. Under these circumstances, the determination of simultaneous urinary clearances of proteins of graded size has been used to characterize the permselective properties of the diseased glomerulus.[20,21] Five or six proteins, which are dispersed over a molecular weight range of 70,000 to 750,000, have usually been studied.

The smallest protein in the series, usually albumin or transferrin (which have Stokes radii of 36 and 38 Å, respectively) is used as a reference marker. The clearance ratio of the larger test proteins to that of the reference protein is then plotted as a function of molecular weight using log–log coordinates. In general, an inverse relationship between this clearance ratio and molecular weight has been observed. This has been interpreted to indicate that the diseased glomerulus continues to discriminate among proteins of increasing size. According to this interpretation, the glomerular size-selective barrier to macromolecule filtration in patients with the nephrotic syndrome differs from that in normal subjects in that its pore size distribution is shifted to pores of larger size than normal. The slope of the regression line that describes the inverse relationship between the test-to-reference protein clearance ratio and molecular weight has been used to evaluate the extent to which glomerular pore size distribution is shifted to pores of larger size. In general, two broad categories of proteinuria may be identified with this technique. These have been designated selective and nonselective, respectively. With the former, a steep slope (often with the shape of a dog's leg) indicates that the membrane has a relatively sharp cut-off, and excreted protein in the urine is composed almost exclusively of the relatively small albumin molecule. With the latter, larger plasma proteins, (the most copious of which is IgG) constitute a substantial fraction of excreted protein.

Instead of determining the concentration in urine and plasma of multiple plasma proteins to construct a differential protein clearance profile, it has been shown that similar information can be obtained by simply determining the clearance ratio of a single large protein (usually IgG) to that of a smaller protein (usually albumin or transferrin). When this clearance ratio, known as the selectivity index, exceeds 0.2, proteinuria is termed nonselective. Conversely a selectivity index of less than 0.2 indicates highly selective proteinuria.[22]

Two major theoretical disadvantages of the differential protein clearance technique limit its usefulness for evaluating the size-selective properties of the glomerular filter.

First, as discussed earlier, there is now abundant evidence to indicate a functionally important interaction between circulating charged macromolecules and anionic components of the glomerular capillary wall.[23] Some of the test proteins employed in determining the selectivity index behave as polyanions in physiological solution, whereas others are neutral or even slightly cationic. Thus, whereas it is now apparent that the glomerulus behaves as a charge-selective as well as a size-selective filter, the differential protein clearance technique as originally conceived has failed to take the former property of the glomerular filtration barrier into account.

Second, the urinary clearance of any protein is a function not only of its filtration rate but also of the rate at which it is reabsorbed from the tubule. When glomerular disease results in only a modest increase in protein filtration into Bowman's space, reabsorption may be in excess of excretion. Under these conditions, the increase in urinary protein excretion is likely to be small, and the relative urinary clearance of graded proteins will be subject to considerable analytical error and hence unsuitable for interpreting events in Bowman's space. With severe glomerular disease, the transglomerular passage of proteins may be considerably enhanced with the result that the capacity of the tubule to take up filtered protein becomes saturated, and urinary protein excretion reaches massive proportions. Under these conditions, the urinary clearance of a given protein may approach its filtration rate.[4, 5] The attribution of differences in clearances among test proteins to altered glomerular permeability, however, requires that the reabsorbed fraction of each filtered protein be constant. Although indirect evidence points to a common tubular reabsorption process for all large proteins,[24] differential protein clearances and the selectivity index as currently employed assume fractional reabsorption to be identical for all proteins. Recent experimental evidence suggests that this assumption may not be justified; thus, inferences regarding glomerular permeability based on urinary protein clearances must remain suspect.[25]

Fractional Dextran Clearances

As discussed earlier, the foregoing limitations of endogenous proteins as transport probes can be avoided with the use of inert and polydisperse polymer macromolecules such as dextran, which are uncharged and are neither reabsorbed nor secreted by the tubule. In the hope that the signficance of the selectivity of proteinuria might be elucidated, there follows an analysis that attempts (1) to interpret changes in transglomerular dextran transport in terms of alterations in membrane pore structure and (2) to relate such dextran transport changes to the selectivity of proteinuria.

The findings of 70 patients referred consecutively to the Stanford University Nephrology Clinic because of nephrotic-range proteinuria are reviewed. The glomerular diseases underlying the development of the nephrotic syndrome were of diverse etiology and varying histopathology and are listed in Table II. Each patient was infused with 130 mg/kg of dextran 40 and 36 mg/kg of inulin. The extent to which the diseased GCW limited the transmural passage of dextran macromolecules as well as those of the endogenous proteins albumin and IgG was determined by comparing the clearance of each macromolecule with that of freely permeable inulin. Assay of dextran in plasma and urine was performed after component dextran molecules (radius interval 20–60 Å) were separated into narrow fractions by gel permeation chromatography on precalibrated Sephacryl S300 columns. As stated previously, rates of reabsorption and secretion of dextran by the renal tubule are negligible; its fractional clearance (relative to inulin) therefore is equivalent to its sieving coefficient, Θ.[7] For purposes of the following analysis, it is assumed that at the high filtered protein loads typical of the nephrotic syndrome, fractional reabsorption of albumin and IgG are minor or negligible and that their fractional clearances approach their respective sieving coefficients.[5]

Theoretical calculations (based on fractional clearances of neutral dextrans) indicate that the normal GCW behaves to good approximation as an isoporous filter with a pore radius of 50–55 Å.[11, 12] It is theoretically possible, therefore, that albumin ($r = 36$ Å) could gain access to Bowman's space in nephrotic subjects because of loss of electrostatic retarda-

Table II. Nephrotic Population Classified by
Etiology and Barrier Injury Grade

	Number of patients			
	Grade 1	Grade 2	Grade 3	Total
Proliferative nephritis	6	10	6	22
Diabetic glomerulopathy	5	10	7	22
Membranous glomerulopathy	5	2	2	9
Amyloidosis	1	2	2	5
Minimal change nephropathy	5	0	0	5
Focal glomerular sclerosis	1	4	2	7

tion by a GCW depleted of its fixed negatively charged components. In contrast, the large size of IgG ($r = 55$ Å) makes it likely that its leakage into Bowman's space, and hence into urine, is a function of the extent to which the size-selective properties of the GCW have become impaired. In the hope that the transglomerular passage of IgG might reflect impaired size selectivity in an unambiguous fashion, the fractional clearance of IgG rather than albumin is used to characterize injury to the filtration barrier in the nephrotic population. Fractional IgG clearance is plotted as a function of the conventional proteinuria selectivity index (C_{IgG}/C_{alb}) in Fig. 3. As shown, there was considerable variability among nephrotic patients in the extent to which the GCW had become hyperpermeable to IgG with the result that fractional IgG clearance spanned three orders of magnitude. Each order of magnitude was arbitrarily used to define the following three grades of progressive barrier injury: grade I, 0.0001–0.001; grade II, 0.001–0.01; grade III, 0.01–0.1.

As can be clearly seen in Fig. 3, minor rates of IgG leakage (grade 1) were associated with a low selectivity index, indicating that although the GCW was highly permeable to albumin, it remained relatively impermeable to IgG. At the opposite extreme (grade III), high rates of IgG leakage were associated with a high selectivity index approaching unity, a finding that is taken to indicate that the GCW discriminated little between the smaller albumin and larger IgG molecule. It is noteworthy that with the exception of minimal-change nephropathy, which was always associated with a low selectivity index, the selectivity index had no predictive value in distinguishing the various categories of glomerulopathy depicted in Table II. Moreover, if focal glomerular sclerosis is regarded as a progressive and advanced form of minimal-change nephropathy, it becomes apparent that all glomerular diseases may exhibit a wide range of selectivity of proteinuria. The magnitude of the selectivity index may in fact represent a nonspecific measure of the

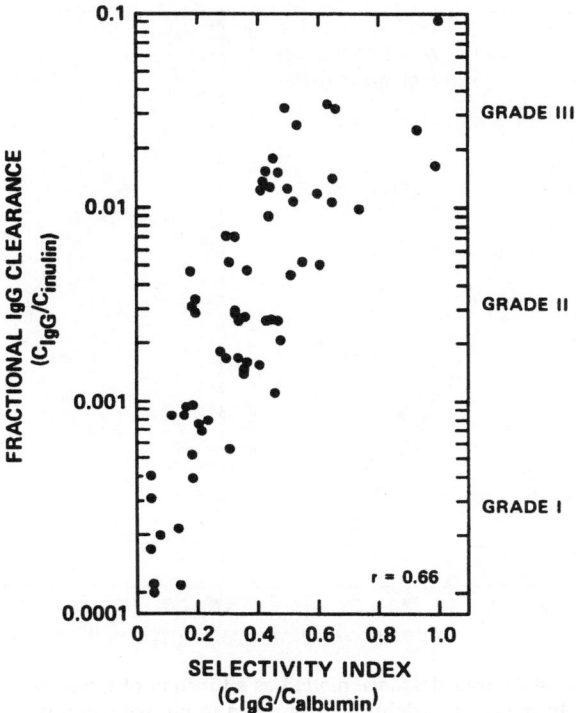

Figure 3. Fractional IgG clearance plotted as a function of the selectivity index in 70 nephrotic patients.

severity of a given glomerular disease. That this is so is suggested by a strong inverse relationship between the fractional IgG clearance and GFR in the two largest categories of patients, namely, those with glomerulonephritis[26] and those with diabetic glomerulopathy.[27] Of interest, the same inverse relationship also holds true when minimal-change nephropathy and focal glomerular sclerosis are regarded as a single entity.

The alteration in size-selective barrier function that underlies the progressive escape of IgG into urine is elucidated by the fractional dextran clearance profiles of each injury grade (Fig. 4). Thus, with grade I injury, Θ for dextrans was restricted over the entire range of molecular sized examined relative to that in the previously described control population of 20 normal volunteers. According to transport theory, this finding implies that glomerular pores in grade I nephrotics are reduced either in size or in number. At first glance, a defect in the charge rather

Bryan D. Myers

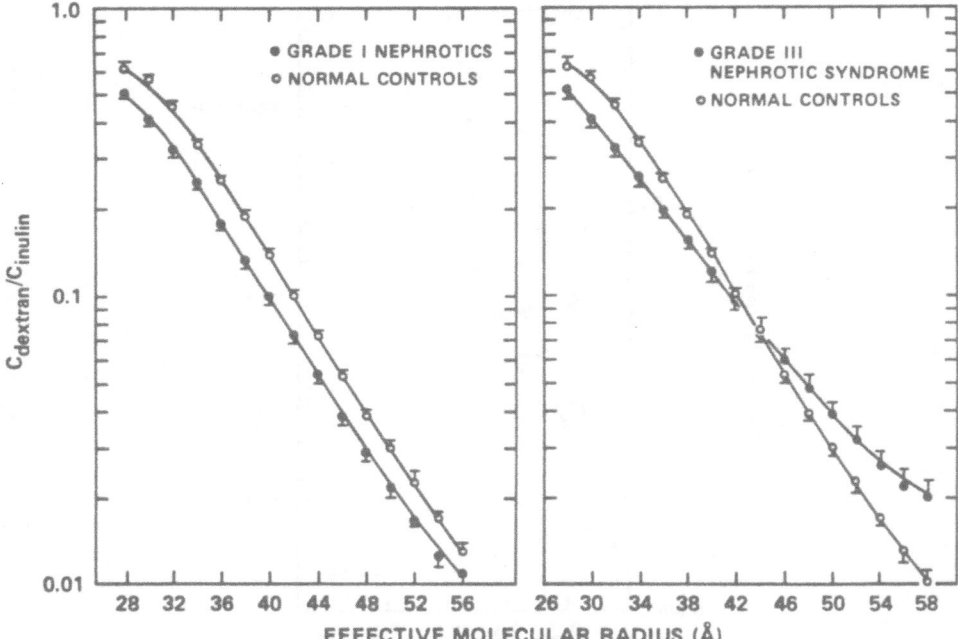

Figure 4. Fractional dextran clearance plotted as a function of molecular radius. Grade I (left) and grade III nephrotics (right) are compared to normal controls.

than size-selective properties of the glomerular filter would appear to be responsible for the rather selective albuminuria. The fractional dextran clearance profile was strikingly different with grades II and III nephrotic injury (Fig. 4, right panel). The Θ of smaller dextrans was once again depressed below normal. For dextrans with radii larger than 54 Å in grade II (not shown) and larger than 44 Å in grade III, however (Fig. 4), Θ was elevated above controls. Moreover, the extent of the enhanced transglomerular transport of large dextrans was magnified with increasing size of the permeating molecule. These findings are inconsistent with an isoporous filter. No single population of pores of identical size can simultaneously account for restricted transport of smaller dextrans and enhanced transport of larger dextrans. Rather, it is now necessary to postulate a heteroporous membrane that contains a subset of pores that are sufficiently large to account for the selective increase in Θ for large, near-impermeant dextran molecules. The same subpopulation of large pores presumably provides the portal of entry for IgG (and probably for most of the filtered albumin load) into Bowman's space.

The heteroporous nature of the GCW becomes clearer when the fractional dextran clearance profiles are plotted on log-normal probability coordinates. In the normal volunteer population, the variation between Θ of dextran and molecular radius on these coordinates is linear, indicating that the normal GCW is composed of a single population of pores with a log–normal and rather narrow distribution of sizes (left panel, Fig. 5). In the three nephrotic groups, by contrast, the fractional dextran clearance profile is curvilinear because of an elevation of the large-radius portion of the profile above linearity. The latter finding is most marked in grade III nephrotics (right panel, Fig. 5), moderate in grade II nephrotics (not shown), and slight in grade I nephrotics (middle panel, Fig. 5). This departure from linearity on log–normal probability coordinates implies that the pores in the nephrotic glomerulus no longer have a single, narrow distribution of pore sizes.

For the sake of simplicity, we have treated the GCW as a heteroporous membrane with a bimodal pore-size distribution. Two mathematical models were devised, both of which interpret the changes in dextran filtration in terms of a parallel array of two radically different pore-structure components. The main component behaves as a small-pore ultrafilter that is responsible for the retention of dextrans with small effective radii. The minor component is postulated to be a large-pore ultrafilter through which large macromolecules (including albumin, IgG, and large dextrans) are able to penetrate. It is this large-pore region that is the defective region of the membrane. The two models differ in that one treats the two membrane arrays as two continuous distributions of pores.[27] The other is a modification of the isoporous model of Deen to the case of a membrane with two discrete pore radii.[26] Both models reveal the major, small-pore component of the membrane in nephrotic subjects to have a distribution of pore size similar to that in the healthy GCW. The minor, large-pore region of the nephrotic glomerular membrane, by contrast, has pore dimensions that would render it permeable to IgG. These enlarged pores are estimated to occupy no more than 6% of the total membrane-pore area, even in the most extreme cases of loss of glomerular size selectivity.

Mechanisms of Glomerular Proteinuria

The foregoing analysis suggests that nephrotic range proteinuria is caused by an alteration of membrane-pore structure. This takes the form of the development of a small subpopulation of enlarged, protein-permeable pores, or defects, within the diseased GCW. It points to loss of size selectivity rather than of charge selectivity as the proximate cause

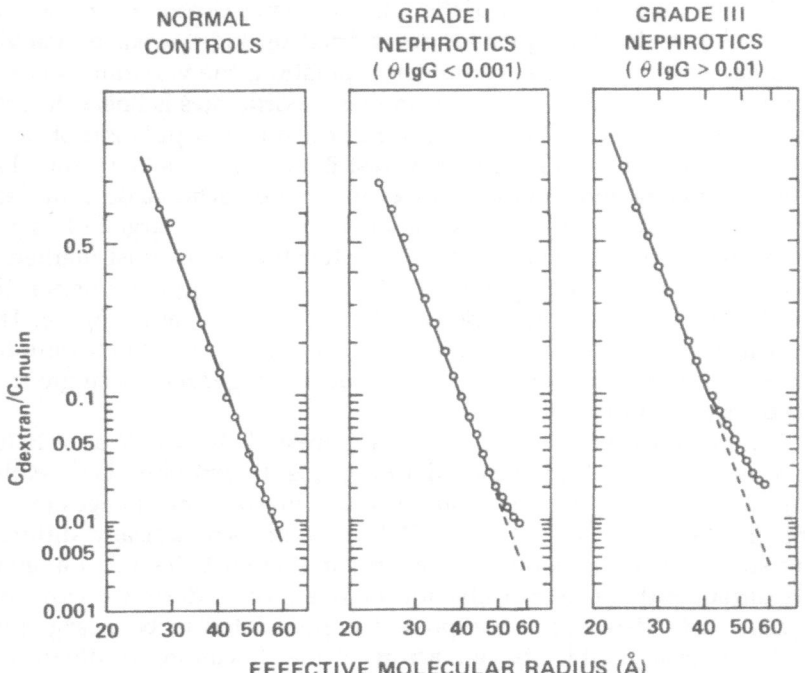

Figure 5. The variation between fractional dextran clearance and dextran radius has been plotted on log–normal probability coordinates. In normal controls the relationship is linear, suggesting a single distribution of pore sizes. The departure from linearity of the large radius part of the dextran sieving curve in nephrotics (middle and right panels) is taken to reflect a bimodal pore-size distribution.

of massive glomerular proteinuria in man. The theoretical analysis from which the membrane parameters consistent with a bimodal pore-size distribution have been derived should not be regarded as a representation of glomerular morphology. Nevertheless, it is interesting to note that a ubiquitous injury that might cause a focal disruption of the glomerular filtration barrier has been observed in several proteinuric glomerulopathies in experimental animals.[28, 29] This injury is characterized by a focal foot process degeneration with detachment of epithelial cells from and denudation of the underlying glomerular basement membrane. Where electron-dense tracers have been injected, they have been observed to penetrate the glomerular basement membrane at these denuded sites exclusively and to enter Bowman's space via the abnormal space beneath the detached epithelial layer.[28,29]

Although a similar injury has been reported in proteinuric man with either diabetic glomerulopathy or focal glomerular sclerosis, such reports are rare.[30] It may be that the shift of glomerular pore-size distribution toward pores of larger size in nephrotic man is not resolvable by conventional electron microscopy. On the other hand, cytochemical techniques reveal that fixed negatively charged components of the glomerular capillary wall are depleted severely in virtually all proteinuric disorders of man.[31] It is conceivable that these polyanionic components, particularly the glycosamine glycans of the basement membrane, determine the distribution and size of pores in the hydrated interior of the matrix of the GCW. Thus, GCW charge depletion resulting from a given glomerulopathy may contribute to proteinuria primarily by altering the size-selective properties of the matrix of the filtration barrier, and any accompanying loss of electrostatic barrier function may play, at most, only a secondary and minor role.[32]

This latter conclusion may apply only in the case of nonminimal glomerulopathies, however. Among the patients with grade I nephrotic injury in the above-described nephrotic population, transglomerular transport of dextrans, including those of large radius, was most restricted in those with minimal change nephropathy. Convincing evidence of loss of size selectivity in this latter entity remains to be demonstrated.[11] Conceivably, minimal-change nephropathy is unique among glomerular diseases in that it represents a pure electrochemical disorder of the GCW and in that the selective albuminuria that typifies it is a consequence of an isolated impairment of electrostatic barrier function.[33]

ACKNOWLEDGMENT. The human data reported in this chapter derive from a study supported by a grant (AM 29985) from the National Institutes of Health.

REFERENCES

1. Deen WM, Robertson CR, Brenner BM: Transcapillary fluid exchange in the renal cortex. Circ Res 33:1–8, 1973
2. Brenner BM, Hostetter TH, Hulmes HD: Glomerular permselectivity: Barrier function based on discrimination of molecular size and charge. Am J Physiol 234:F455–F460, 1978
3. Harris CA, Baer PG, Chirito R, et al: Composition of mammalian glomerular filtrate. Am J Physiol 227:972–976, 1974
4. Galaske RG, Van Liew JB, Field LG: Filtration and reabsorption of endogenous low-molecular-weight protein in the rat kidney. Kidney Int 16:394–403, 1979
5. Oken DE, Kirschbaum BB, Landwehr DM: Micropuncture studies of the mechanisms of normal and pathologic albuminuria, in Berlyne GM (ed): Contribution to Nephrology, vol 24. Basel, S Karger, 1981, pp. 1–7

6. Rennke HG, Patel Y, Venkatachalam MA: Glomerular filtration of proteins: Clearances of anionic, neutral and cationic horseradish peroxidase in the rat. *Kidney Int* 13:324–328, 1978
7. Chang RLS, Ueki IF, Troy JL, et al: Permselectivity of the glomerular capillary wall to macromolecules. II. Experimental studies in rats using neutral dextran. *Biophys J* 15:887–895, 1975
8. Gassee JP, Dubois R, Staroukine M, et al: Determination of glomerular intracapillary and transcapillary pressure gradients from sieving data: III. The effects of angiotensin II. *Pfluegers Arch* 367:15–26, 1976
9. Hardwicke J, Hulme B, Jones JH, et al: Measurement of glomerular permeability to polydisperse radioactivity labelled macromolecules in normal rabbits. *Clin Sci* 34:505–514, 1968
10. Pappenheimer JR, Renkin EM, Borrero LM: Filtration, diffusion and molecular sieving through peripheral capillary membranes. A contribution to the pore theory of capillary permeability. *Am J Physiol* 167:13–46, 1951
11. Winetz JA, Robertson CR, Golbetz H, et al: The nature of the glomerular injury in minimal change and focal sclerosing glomerulopathies. *Am J Kidney Dis* 1:91–98, 1981
12. Deen WM, Myers BD, Brenner BM: The glomerular barrier to macromolecules: Theoretical and experimental considerations, in Brenner BM (ed): *Contemporary Issues in Nephrology: Nephrotic Syndrome.* New York, Churchill Livingstone, 1982, pp. 1–29
13. Bohrer MP, Bayliss C, Humes HD, et al: Permselectivity of the glomerular capillary wall. Facilitated filtration of circulating polycations. *J Clin Invest* 61:72–78, 1978
14. Deen WM, Satvat B, Jamieson JM: Theoretical model for glomerular filtration of charged solutes. *Am J Physiol* 238:F126–F139, 1980
15. Venkatachalam MA, Rennke HG: The structural and molecular basis of glomerular filtration. *Circ Res* 43:337–347, 1978
16. Schneeberger EE, Levey RH, McCluskey RT, et al: The isoporous substructure of the human glomerular slit diaphragm. *Kidney Int* 8:48–52, 1975
17. Rennke HG, Venkatachalam MA: Glomerular permeability: In vivo tracer studies with polyanionic and polycationic ferritins. *Kidney Int.* 11:44–53, 1977
18. Kanwar YS, Farquhar MG: Anionic sites in the glomerular basement membrane. In vivo and in vitro localization to the laminae rarae by cationic probes. *J Cell Biol* 81:137–153, 1979
19. Latta H, Johnston WH: The glycoprotein inner layer of glomerular capillary basement membrane as a filtration barrier. *J Ultrastruct Res* 57:65–67, 1976
20. Joachim GR, Cameron JS, Schartz M: Selectivity of protein excretion in patients with the nephrotic syndrome. *J Clin Invest* 43:2332–2346, 1964
21. Hardwicke J, Cameron JS, Harrison JF: Proteinuria studied by clearances of individual macromolecules. In Manuel Y, Revillard JP (eds): *Proteins in Normal and Pathological Urine.* University Park Press, Baltimore, 1970, p 128
22. Cameron JS, Blandford G: The simple assessment of selectivity in heavy proteinuria. *Lancet* 2:242–247, 1966
23. Deen WM, Satvat B: Determinants of the glomerular filtration of proteins. *Am J Physiol* 10:F162–F170, 1981
24. Hardwicke J, Squire JR: The relationship between plasma albumin concentration and protein excretion in patients with proteinuria. *Clin Sci* 14:509–530, 1955
25. Christensen EI, Rennke HG, Carone FA: Renal tubular uptake of protein: Effect of molecular charge. *Am J Physiol* 244:F436–F441, 1983
26. Myers BD, Okarma TB, Friedman S, et al: Mechanisms of proteinuria in human glomerulonephritis. *J Clin Invest* 70:732–746, 1982

27. Myers BD, Winetz JA, Chui F, et al: Mechanisms of proteinuria in diabetic nephropathy: A study of glomerular barrier function. *Kidney Int* 21:96–105, 1982
28. Olson JL, Rennke HG, Venkatachalam MA: Alterations in the charge and size selectivity barrier of the gomerular filter in aminonuscleoside nephrosis in rats. *Lab Invest* 44:271–279, 1981
29. Olson JL, Hostetter TH, Rennke HG, et al: Altered glomerular permselectivity and progressive sclerosing following extreme ablation of renal mass. *Kidney Int* 22:112–126, 1982
30. Cohen AH, Mampaso F, Zamboni L: Glomerular podocyte degeneration in human renal disease. An ultrastructural study. *Lab Invest* 37:30–42, 1977
31. Blau EB, Haas DE: Glomerular sialic acid and proteinuria in human renal disease. *Lab Invest* 28:477–488, 1973
32. Kanwar YS, Rosenzweig LJ: Altered glomerular permeability as a result of focal detachment of the visceral epithelium. *Kidney Int* 21:565–574, 1982
33. Bridges CR, Myers BD, Brenner B, et al: Glomerular charge alterations in human minimal change nephropathy. *Kidney Int* 22:677–684, 1982

3

Tubular Handling of Proteins

Absorption of Albumin by Isolated Perfused Proximal Convoluted Tubules of the Rabbit

C. HYUNG PARK, MARIA JOSE F. CAMARGO,
AND THOMAS MAACK

INTRODUCTION

The glomerular apparatus provides an effective, albeit not absolute, barrier against the filtration of larger plasma proteins such as albumin and globulins. The small amounts of these proteins that gain access to the glomerular filtrate are almost completely absorbed by the tubular epithelium. Tubular handling assumes a greater significance when glomerular permselectivity is altered and significant amounts of larger proteins, particularly albumin, are filtered. Under these conditions, the kidneys may play an important role in the overall disposal of circulating albumin. Unfortunately, in view of the technical difficulties in the quantitation of basic parameters such as the concentration of albumin in the glomerular filtrate, very little is known about the kinetics of the tubular uptake of albumin and the further fate of the absorbed protein.

On the other hand, a great deal has been learned about the general process of tubular absorption and catabolism of low-molecular-weight proteins. These proteins, which are extensively filtered by the kidney, constitute a small but biologically important fraction of the total protein mass and comprise a variety of biologically active principles including proteohormones (e.g., insulin, PTH, growth hormone), enzymes (e.g., lysozyme), immunoprotein fragments (e.g., Bence Jones protein), and membrane antigens (e.g., β_2-microglobulin).

C. HYUNG PARK, MARIA JOSE F. CAMARGO, AND THOMAS MAACK • Department of Physiology, Cornell University Medical College, New York, New York 10021.

In the present chapter we consider the process of tubular absorption and catabolism of proteins in general and of albumin in particular. For this purpose we briefly summarize the evidence obtained in our laboratory regarding the tubular processing of low-molecular-weight proteins[1,2] and then describe in more detail our recent study on the absorption and catabolism of albumin by isolated perfused proximal convoluted tubules of the rabbit kidney.[3]

ENDOCYTIC UPTAKE OF PROTEINS BY RENAL CELLS

Studies on tubular absorption and catabolism of proteins came initially from the quest to understand on one hand the fascinating process of cell uptake and hydrolysis of proteins and, on the other hand, to gain insights into the pathophysiology of proteinurias. Furthermore, in the last two decades, it became apparent that the kidney plays a major role in the disposal and regulation of plasma levels of low-molecular-weight proteins (LMWP).[1,2] Oliver and colleagues,[4,5] in studies spanning five decades, provided systematic evidence that the "hyaline droplets" present in renal cells of proteinuric kidneys are in reality protein absorption droplets rather than simple images of cell degeneration, as initially thought. These studies opened the field of protein transport and catabolism by renal tubular cells.

The elegant work of Werner Straus in the 1950s and 1960s pioneered our understanding of the general mechanisms of these processes.[6-8] In a series of incisive experiments using morphological and differential centrifugation techniques and introducing horseradish peroxidase as a probe protein, Straus described the endocytic uptake of proteins by renal tubular cells. His description, with small refinements, is now accepted by all investigators as the universal process by which not only renal cells but all cells of the body dispose of absorbed proteins. Figure 1 presents a schematic view of this process. Proteins are internalized into the renal cells by endocytosis, a phenomenon that is particularly prominent on the luminal side of proximal tubule cells. Then the endocytic vesicle containing the absorbed protein migrates to the cell's interior and eventually fuses with lysosomes, the cell organelles that contain acid hydrolases capable of catabolizing proteins. This event, and the observation that absorbed proteins are no longer visible in the cell interior after a certain period of time, led Straus to postulate that absorbed proteins are hydrolyzed within these cell organelles. The general features of the endocytic process as described by Straus were fully confirmed by several laboratories.[9-13] It was further demonstrated that the hydrolysis of absorbed

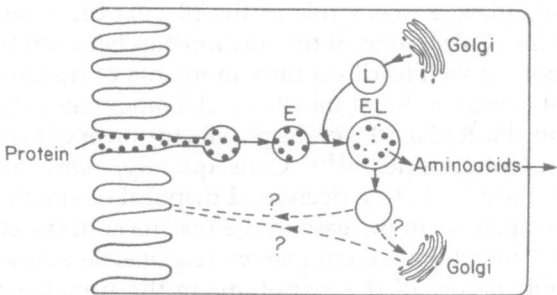

Figure 1. Schematic representation of the endocytic uptake of filtered proteins. Proteins are adsorbed to binding sites at the luminal membrane and segregated in endosomes (E). The endsomes then migrate to the cell interior where they fuse with lysosomes (L). Digestion of the protein takes place within the endolysosomes (EL). The resulting amino acids are then delivered to the circulation across the peritubular cell membrane. The fate of the "empty" endolysosome is unknown, but it may fuse with other endocytic vesicles or lysosomes, migrate to the Golgi apparatus, or fuse with the luminal membrane. (From Maack et al.[2] with permission from Raven Press.)

protein goes to completion and that the resulting amino acids are returned to the circulation via the peritubular side.[1,2,14–16]

RENAL HANDLING OF LOW-MOLECULAR-WEIGHT PROTEINS

Most of the earlier studies on protein handling by the kidney were qualitative or semiquantitative in nature. In the past decade, quantitative physiological studies led to a better, albeit still incomplete, understanding of the process of renal extraction, filtration, tubular absorption, and renal metabolism of LMWP under normal and pathological conditions. A brief description of the main conclusions of these studies is given below. For a more complete overview and detailed bibliographic references, the reader is directed to recent reviews on the subject.[1,2]

Circulating low-molecular-weight proteins gain access to the renal cells mainly by the filtration route. The amount of protein filtered is directly proportional to the GFR, the plasma concentration of the protein, and its glomerular sieving coefficient. The latter is predominantly determined by the size of the low-molecular-weight protein and is usually greater than 0.5[1,2] for the most important circulating small proteins and proteohormones. This leads to daily filtered loads that are many times larger than the plasma pool of these proteins. Since, as is discussed below, filtered proteins are eventually hydrolyzed by tubular cells, the kidney plays a major role in the plasma turnover of circulating small proteins. Calculation of the relationship between filtered loads and plasma pools as well as direct measurements of fractional renal extractions (renal extraction/total metabolic clearance rate) show that the kidney is responsible for 30–80% of the plasma turnover of most circulating LMWP and proteohormones.[1,14-18] Consequently, removal of the kidneys or renal failure leads to a decreased disposal of circulating LMWP and for the most part to an increase in the plasma concentration of these substances.[19-25] This phenomenon may be responsible at least in part for the kaleidoscopic nature of the symptoms in the uremic syndrome.

Under normal conditions, filtered proteins are extensively absorbed by the proximal tubular epithelium, with very little appearing in the urine.[1,2,14,17,18,21,26-28] Uptake of proteins is directly or indirectly dependent on cell energy and occurs via an adsorptive endocytic mechanism; i.e., proteins bind to the luminal membrane and/or to the endocytic sites of the luminal membrane before incorporation into the cell.[1,2,14-18] The absorption process is saturable with a high capacity and low affinity compared to the normal filtered loads of LMWP.[14-18,28] These characteristics of tubular absorption imply that spillage of LMWP in urine occurs either because of an impairment of tubular function (tubular proteinurias) or because of an increase in the plasma concentration of a particular LMWP (overload proteinurias). In the latter case, in view of the low affinity of the uptake process, LMWP appear in urine long before the tubular absorption is saturated. Consequently, there is a concomitant increase in urinary excretion and tubular absorption rates over a large range of filtered loads. As a result, in overload proteinurias, there may be deposition of specific LMWP in tubular cells (e.g., Bence Jones proteinuria or lysozymuria[29,30]).

Although there is a clear demonstration that cationic proteins may compete for absorption,[28,31] tubular uptake of LMWP is a selective process.[28] The selectivity is determined by a complex set of parameters that include (1) the physiocochemical nature of the protein molecule such as net charge, type of positively charged groups, size, and compactness, (2) the preferential uptake of some proteins (e.g., β_2-microglobulin) in the initial portions of the proximal tubule, and (3) the complex structural relationship between the microvilli and the endocytic sites at the base of the microvilli, which may determine the degree of access of proteins to the endocytic site. The selectivity of the process of tubular uptake of proteins implies that excess load of a particular LMWP is not necessarily accompanied by an increased urinary excretion of all filtered proteins.

Absorbed LMWP are hydrolyzed to completion within phagolysosomes, and the resulting amino acids are returned to the circulation.[1,2,14-18] In addition to this universal processing of all filtered proteins, small linear peptides (e.g., angiotensin II) are hydrolyzed by brush border proteases,[32] and some proteohormones that have receptors at the peritubular site (e.g., PTH, insulin) are partially hydrolyzed at these sites.[26,27,33] The rate of hydrolysis of absorbed proteins depends on the nature of the protein, the half-time of hydrolysis being of the order of minutes for, e.g., proteohormones and hours or even days for certain endogenous LMWP or injected foreign proteins.[1,2,7,11,15,17] Lysosomal catabolism of poorly hydrolyzable proteins (e.g., lysozyme and probably Bence Jones protein) tends to saturate at high absorption rates of these proteins.[1,2,11] However, there is at least some selectivity of hydrolytic process, since saturation of the intracellular hydrolysis of a particular protein (e.g., cytochrome c) does not interfere with the disposal of another protein (e.g., hGH).[2,34] The acid milieu within the lysosomes is essential for the normal disposal of absorbed protein. Thus, alkalinization of renal cell lysosomes by NH_4Cl or chloroquine reversibly inhibits the hydrolysis of absorbed cytochrome c.[2]

The characteristics of the hydrolytic process of absorbed LMWP imply that the bulk of filtered protein is catabolized by the kidney with a recovery for the organism of the constituent amino acids. The lower the rate constant of hydrolysis of an absorbed protein, the greater will be the tendency for the formation of protein absorption droplets on an increase in its plasma concentration. This may explain in part the tendency for the formation of protein absorption droplets in multiple myeloma (Bence Jones proteinuria)[30] or in myelocytic leukemias (lysozymuria).[29] Protein absorption droplets may also be present at normal filtered loads of protein if there is a defect in lysosomal acidification. Such a defect may occur if the lysosomal membrane permeability to protons is increased and/or if there is a deficient energy supply to the lysosomal proton pump.

TUBULAR ABSORPTION AND CATABOLISM OF ALBUMIN

General Considerations and Methodological Problems

Morphological studies have shown that albumin present in tubular fluid is also endocytosed by renal tubular cells, localized in phagolysosomes, and most probably catabolized within these cell organelles.[10,13] Furthermore, microperfusion experiments in the kidneys of intact rats demonstrate that the bulk of albumin absorption takes place in the proximal convoluted tubule.[35] Interest in the study of tubular absorption of albumin has been fueled by the fact that this is the most abundant of the plasma proteins and that albuminuria and hypoalbuminemia are such prevalent features in many renal diseases. In contrast, however, to the relatively large body of evidence regarding the renal processing of LMWP summarized above, very little is known about the quantitative aspects of the tubular absorption and catabolism of albumin. This is not entirely surprising, since the quantitation of the tubular uptake of albumin encounters considerable technical difficulties.

The major methodological problems in studying the quantitative aspects of tubular absorption and catabolism of albumin may be summarized as follows: (1) in view of the very low glomerular sieving coefficient of albumin, whole-organ clearance methods are entirely inadequate to quantitate the tubular absorption of this protein; (2) the measurement of the very small concentrations of albumin in the nanoliter samples of glomerular filtrate or tubular fluid obtained in micropuncture experiments is still rather imprecise even with the use of very sensitive immunologic procedures; (3) the contamination of tubular fluid poor in albumin with extraluminal fluid rich in albumin may lead to an overestimation of albumin concentration in glomerular filtrate or tubular fluid samples; and (4) the strong and dose-dependent binding of albumin even to siliconized micropipettes may lead to an underestimation of the concentration of this protein in tubular fluid samples.

The difficulties enumerated above led to disagreements among investigators about the values of even such a basic parameter as the normal concentration of albumin in the glomerular filtrate. Thus, although it is generally agreed that the mean albumin concentration in the filtrate is less than 3 and possibly less than 1 mg/dl, the reported values may scatter over a range of tenfold or more even in micropuncture samples obtained by the same group of investigators in a single animal.[36-44] This scatter is still larger in proteinuric models,[38,39,41,42,44] in which, in addition to the above mentioned methodological problems, there is certainly a large heterogeneity of glomerular permselectivities among different nephrons in the same animal. The large variability of the measurements of tubular fluid albumin concentrations precludes a precise quantitation of the kinetics of albumin absorption. Nevertheless, based on micropuncture studies comparing albumin absorption in normal and proteinuric rats, several investigators claim that, in contrast to what has been demonstrated for low-molecular-weight proteins, albumin absorption saturates at near normal filtered loads of this protein.[38-44]

Methods of Determining Albumin Transport and Catabolism in
Isolated Perfused Proximal Convoluted Tubules of the Rabbit Kidney

Recently, we undertook a study to investigate the quantitative aspects of tubular absorption and catabolism of albumin using techniques that circumvent the technical difficulties described above.[3] For this purpose, isolated proximal convoluted tubules of the rabbit were perfused according to a slight modification of the technique developed by Burg and co-workers.[45,46] The use of the isolated tubule preparation allowed for the establishment of known parameters such as tubular fluid albumin concentrations and loads and in this manner permitted the precise determination of the tubular uptake rates under a variety of conditions and within a large range of concentrations of the protein. Albumin binding to the siliconized glass micropipettes used in the perfusion system was avoided by precoating these pipettes with protein. Under these conditions, recovery of albumin at concentrations as low as 0.0046 mg/ml was greater than 95% and not significantly different from 100%.[3] Finally, to avoid the problem of measuring very low concentrations of albumin by chemical or immunologic methods, we labeled pure crystalline bovine albumin with ^{3}H by the reductive methylation pocedure of Tack *et al.*[47] This method leads to very high specific activies (about 200 Ci/mmol) without affecting the physicochemical or biological activities of proteins. Gel chromatographic and isoelectric focusing determinations showed that the labeled albumin could not be differentiated from the unlabeled protein. The use of labeled albumin had the added advantage that the fate of the absorbed albumin (intracellular accumulation, catabolism, transport of intact protein across the epithelium, nonspecific leak) could also be determined with precision. The main disadvantage of the methodology, as in any *in vitro* preparation, is that the quantitative results should not be automatically extrapolated to intact experimental animals or humans. For details of the methodology, the reader is directed to reference 3.

General Characteristics of the
Tubular Absorption and Catabolism of Albumin

Figure 2 shows the results of the determinations of the tubular absorption and fate of absorbed ^{3}H$_3$C-albumin in tubules perfused with an albumin concentration of 0.03 mg/ml. This concentration is in the upper range of physiological values reported in the mammalian glomerular filtrate.[36-44] The results illustrated in panel A demonstrate that, as ex-

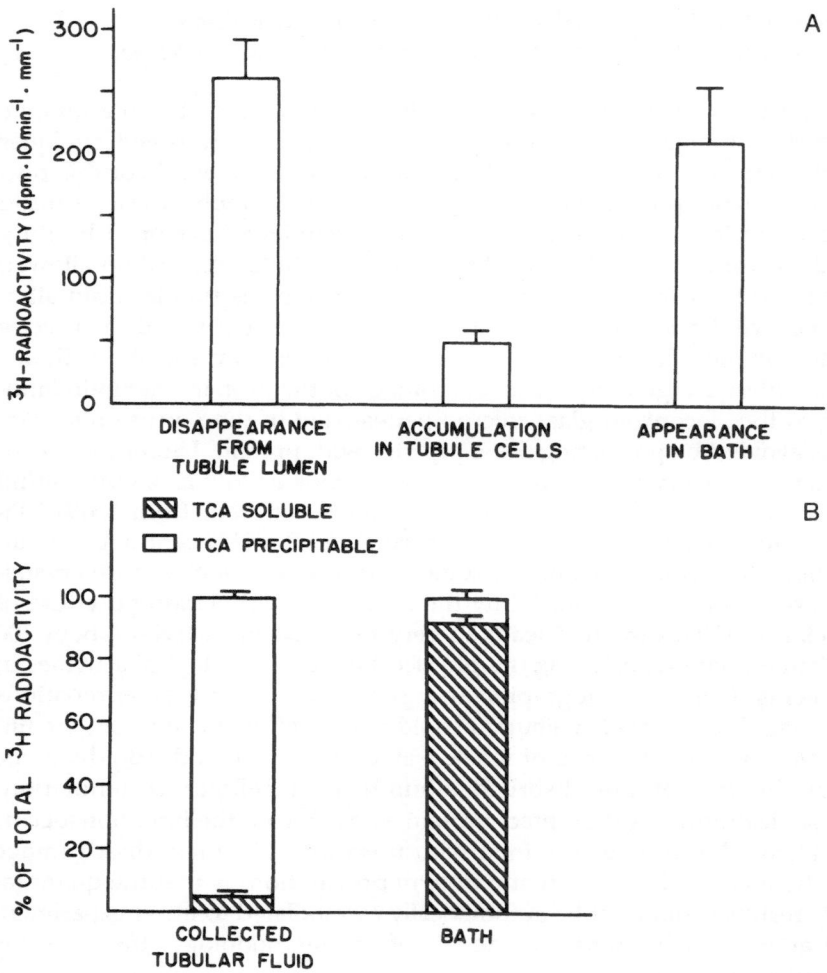

Figure 2. Fate of luminal fluid ^3H_3C-albumin in proximal convoluted tubules of the rabbit. Six tubules were perfused with an albumin concentration of 0.03 mg/ml for about 2h. Total and trichloroacetic acid (TCA)-soluble ^3H radioactivity were determined in the perfusate, collected tubular fluid, and bathing solution. The radioactivity remaining in the tubular tissue at the end of perfusion was also determined. A: The bulk of the radioactivity that disappears from the tubular lumen (about 80%) appears in the bathing solution, with very little of the absorbed radioactivity (about 20%) remaining in the tubular tissue. Results are expressed as mean ± S.E. B: Corresponding values (mean ± SE) for the TCA-soluble and TCA-precipitable radioactivity in the collected perfusion fluid and in the bathing solution. Almost all of the radioactivity in collected tubular fluid is TCA precipitable, showing that the label remains attached to albumin in the fluid. In contrast, almost all of the radioactivity that appears in the bathing solution is TCA soluble, showing that the absorbed ^3H_3C-albumin is catabolized by the tubular epithelium and that the hydrolytic products are delivered to the bathing solution. (From Park and Maack[3] with permission.)

pected, the disappearance of ^3H radioactivity from the tubular lumen (measured by the difference between its perfused and collected loads) is nearly equal to the sum of radioactivity appearing in the bathing solution (measured by the ^3H counts in the bathing solution) and that remaining in tubular tissue. The data depicted in panel B show that the radioactivity in the collected tubular fluid was almost all precipitated by trichloroacetic acid (TCA), demonstrating that there is no dissociation of the label in the tubular fluid. On the other hand, the ^3H radioactivity appearing in the bathing solution was practically all TCA soluble, demonstrating that the absorbed protein is catabolized by the tubular epithelium and that the catabolites are delivered to the peritubular bathing solution. Since practically no intact ^3H_3C-albumin appears in the bathing solution, nonspecific leaks and transcellular transport of intact albumin is negligible or nonexistent. Of note is the finding that very little of the absorbed albumin (about 20%) remained accumulated in tubular tissue by the end of perfusion (panel A, Fig. 2). This indicates that, at least at low loads, the rate of intracellular hydrolysis of albumin parallels its rate of absorption and that accumulation of albumin in renal cells grossly underestimates the true rate of absorption of the protein. The results as a whole demonstrate that the rate of disappearance of ^3H from the tubular lumen is a true measure of the rate of absorption of albumin.

Effect of Iodoacetate on Tubular Absorption of Albumin

Tubular absorption of low-molecular-weight proteins is blocked by several metabolic inhibitors, including cyanide, high concentrations of iodoacetate (IAA), and anoxia.[1,2,14-18,28] To test whether the same is true for albumin, we measured tubular absorption of this protein before and after the addition of 4 mM of IAA to the bathing solution. Each tubule served as its own control. Figure 3 summarizes the results of these experiments. Iodoacetate almost completely inhibited albumin absorption to $3.9 \pm 5.8\%$ of its value in control periods. As expected, the high IAA concentrations used in these experiments also inhibited fluid reabsorption (J_v). However the inhibition of J_v ($45.4 \pm 8.1\%$ of its value in control periods) was significantly less than that of albumin absorption. Although the effect of other metabolic inhibitors was not tested, these results suggest that albumin absorption, like the uptake of low-molecular-weight proteins, is also directly, or indirectly, dependent on cell energy.

Relationship between Albumin Absorption and Fluid Reabsorption

At low perfusate albumin concentration (0.03 mg/ml), there is a proportionality between albumin absorption and fluid reabsorption that results in a near constancy of the tubular fluid albumin concentration in

C.Hyung Park *et al.*

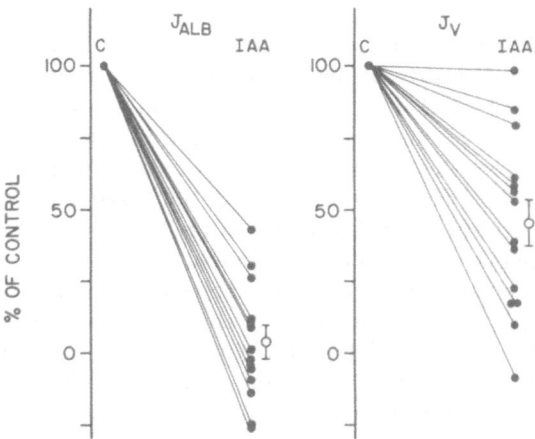

Figure 3. Effect of iodoacetate (IAA) on albumin absorption (J_{ALB}) and fluid reabsorption (J_v) by isolated perfused proximal convoluted tubules of the rabbit. Fourteen tubules were perfused with albumin concentrations from 0.0012 to 2 mg/ml. After control periods (C), 4 mM IAA was added to the bathing solution. Values are expressed as percent of control values (C = 100%). Each individual experiment is represented, and the mean ± S.E. values for all 14 tubules are depicted by the open circles and bars. Iodoacetate almost completely abolished J_{ALB} and significantly decreased J_v. The IAA-induced decrease in J_{ALB} was significantly more pronounced than that of J_v ($P<0.05$). (From Park and Maack[3] with permission.)

the proximal tubule. Indeed, the collected fluid : perfused fluid albumin concentration ratio is 1.02 ± 0.01 ($n = 6$ tubules), a value that is not significantly different from 1.00 ($P>0.05$). This parallelism of albumin absorption and fluid reabsorption has also been reported to occur in proximal tubules of the rat and dog.[36-43] However, protein uptake and fluid reabsorption occur by different mechanisms and can be dissociated. Thus, cytochalasin B, a substance that disrupts microfilaments and may interfere with endocytosis, markedly inhibits the tubular uptake of low-molecular-weight proteins at doses that do not affect fluid reabsorption.[1,28] Furthermore, as shown in the present study, IAA inhibits albumin absorption to a greater extent than J_v, suggesting a dissociation between these two processes.

Definitive proof of this dissociation was obtained in experiments in which albumin absorption and J_v were determined in the presence of chloroquine.[48] Results of these experiments are shown in Fig. 4. Chloroquine (CQ) inhibited the tubular absorption of albumin by a yet unknown mechanism but had no effect on fluid reabsorption. These data demonstrate that there is no tight coupling between the transport of albumin and fluid in the proximal tubule. Whether the parallelism of these

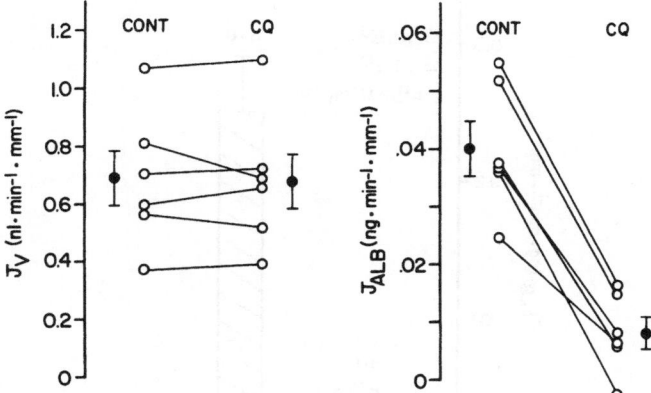

Figure 4. Effect of chloroquine (CQ) on albumin absorption (J_{ALB} and fluid reabsorption (J_v) by isolated perfused proximal convoluted tubules of the rabbit. Six tubules were perfused with an albumin concentration of 0.036 mg/ml. After control periods (CONT), 0.1 mM CQ was added to the bathing solution. Each individual experiment is represented, and the mean ± S.E. values for all six tubules are depicted by the closed circles and bars. Chloroquine markedly decreased J_{ALB} ($P < 0.001$) but had no effect on J_v. Data from Park and Maack.[48]

two processes under normal conditions is simply coincidental or arises from some unknown interaction remains to be elucidated. Equally unknown is the relationship between tubular flow rates and albumin absorption, although some investigators claim that albumin absorption rates depend on contact time.[44] Unfortunately, the present experiments do not help to clarify this issue since the tubules were perfused within a relatively narrow range of flows (10–15 nl/min).

Influence of Net Charge on the Tubular Absorption of Albumin

Previous morphological and quantitative studies indicated that net charge of a protein is one of the determinants of its tubular uptake.[28,41,49,50] To test whether this is also the case for albumin, we compared the tubular absorption of native anionic albumin (pI = 4.6) with that of a derivatized cationic albumin (pI = 8.2). The latter was prepared by amination of carboxyl groups of albumin with ethylenediamine according to the method of Hoare and Koshland.[51] Figure 5 shows that at relatively low concentrations (0.1 mg/ml) cationic albumin is absorbed at about fivefold higher rates than anionic albumin. However, at higher concentrations (>0.4 mg/ml), cationic but not anionic albumin leads to marked abnormalities in tubular functions, significantly depressing fluid reabsorption and protein uptake.[3] This finding in the isolated perfused

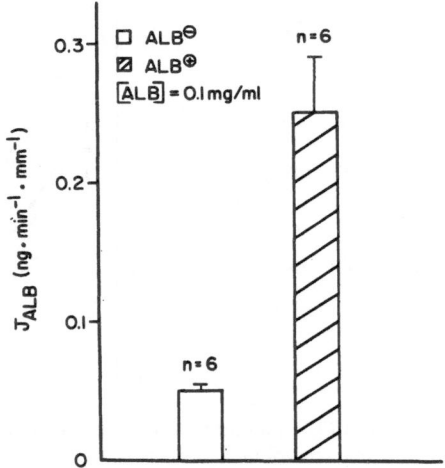

Figure 5. Effect of net charge of albumin on the tubular absorption of albumin by isolated perfused proximal convoluted tubules of the rabbit. Tubules were perfused with 0.1 mg/ml of native anionic albumin (ALB⁻, pI = 4.6) or derivatized cationic albumin (ALB⁺, pI = 8.4). Albumin absorption rates (J_{ALB}) are expressed as mean ± S.E. (n = number of tubules). At this concentration of albumin, the absorption of cationic albumin was about fivefold greater than that of native anionic albumin ($P < 0.01$). At higher concentrations (not shown, see ref. 3), cationic but not anionic albumin markedly depressed fluid and protein transport. Modified from Park and Maack[3] with permission.)

proximal tubule of the rabbit confirms our previous observation in isolated perfused kidneys that high concentrations of strongly cationic compounds such as lysine induce marked morphological damage, particularly in the brush border of proximal convoluted tubules.[28,34]

The demonstration that at low concentration, cationic albumin is absorbed at higher rates than native anionic albumin confirms that net charge is one of the determinants of the tubular uptake of proteins and suggests that binding of albumin to the negatively charged surface of the luminal membrane plays a role in the aborptive process.[50] It should be pointed out, however, that net charge is not the sole and in many conditions not the most important determinant of the tubular uptake of macromolecules, since some highly cationic macromolecules (e.g., cationized dextrans) are not extensively absorbed by the tubular epithelium.[52] The type of positive charge, the size and compactness of the macromolecule, as well as complex structural relationships between microvilli and endocytic sites also may play important roles in the selectivity of the tubular uptake of proteins in general and of albumin in particular.[2,28] These determinants, however, are not yet amenable to quantitative experimentation, and, therefore, their precise role still remains a matter of conjecture.

Kinetics of Tubular Absorption of Albumin

One of the main issues concerning the renal processing of filtered albumin is the relationship between the T_m of absorption and the normal filtered loads of this protein. We have previously shown that for low-molecular-weight proteins the T_m of absorption is far above their normal filtered loads.[1,2,14-18,28] Several investigators have claimed, however, that this is not the case for albumin.[38,39,41-44] We therefore decided to study the kinetics of albumin absorption in isolated perfused proximal convoluted tubules of the rabbit in which perfused loads and absorption rates can be precisely quantitated.[3] For this purpose, we used 57 tubules with albumin concentrations from 0.0012 to 10 mg/ml, a range that encompasses very low physiological to very high pathological albumin concentrations in the glomerular filtrate.

Figure 6 shows the titration curve of albumin absorption as a function of the perfusate concentration of albumin. As can be seen, the overall curve has the classical features of saturation kinetics. The maximal capacity of absorption is reached at tubular fluid concentrations of about 2 mg/ml (V_{max} = 3.7 ng/min per mm tubule length). This is far above the albumin concentration in the filtrate of normal mammalian nephrons. If the length of the proximal convoluted tubule is taken as 6 mm, maximal absorption of albumin by this nephron segment would be about 20 ng/min or about two orders of magnitude greater than the estimated filtered load of albumin in the mammalian kidney. The apparent affinity of the absorption process (apparent K_m = 1.2 mg/ml) is low when compared to the normal concentration of albumin in the filtrate. Below saturation, in the linear range of the absorption curve (Fig. 6), fractional uptake of albumin is relatively constant and amounts to approximately 10% of the load per millimeter tubule length. By the end of 6 mm of proximal convoluted tubule length, this would correspond to about 50–60% of the filtered load of albumin, a value that agrees closely with that derived from micropuncture studies in the intact rat.[37-41,43,44]

Figure 6 (inset) shows that in addition to the overall high-absorptive-capacity system, there is a lower-capacity system with a V_{max} = 0.064 ng/min per mm tubule length and an apparent K_m = 0.031 mg/ml. These values are much closer to the normal albumin concentrations and loads in the mammalian nephron. Therefore, there is a dual kinetics of albumin transport in the isolated perfused proximal convoluted tubule of the rabbit: a high-capacity system that saturates at far above normal and a

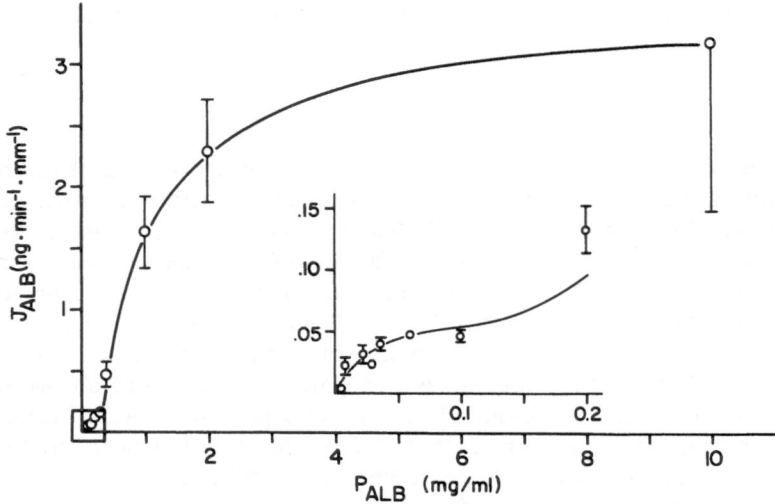

Figure 6. Kinetics of albumin absorption by isolated perfused proximal convoluted tubules of the rabbit. Albumin absorption rates (J_{ALB}) are plotted against the luminal perfusate concentration of albumin (P_{ALB}). Each of 57 tubules was perfused with a fixed P_{ALB} ranging from 0.0012 to 10 mg/ml. Values are mean ± S.E. of at least three tubules. The absorption curve has at least two components: an overall high-capacity, low-affinity system ($J_{ALB}^{max} = 3.7$ ng/min per mm tubule length, apparent $K_m = 1.2$ mg/ml) and a low-capacity system (inset), which saturates near the physiological ranges of tubular fluid concentrations of albumin in mammals ($J_{ALB}^{max} = 0.0064$ ng/min per mm, apparent $K_m = 0.031$ mg/ml). (From Park and Maack[3] with permission.)

low-capacity system that saturates near the normal filtered loads of this protein.

The suggestion that albumin absorption saturates near the normal filtered loads of this protein was derived from micropuncture data comparing albumin absorption in normal rats with that of rats made proteinuric by the administration of aminonucleoside,[38,39] angiotensin,[41] or relatively low doses of anti-GBM antibody.[41-44] Inspection of these data shows that filtrate concentrations of albumin ranged from 0.01 mg/ml in normal rats to about 0.1 mg/ml in proteinuric rats with a very large scatter. These values encompass the operational range of the lower-capacity system described in the present study. Therefore, the failure to detect a high absorptive capacity for albumin may have been attributable to the relatively low tubular fluid albumin concentrations attained in the proteinuric models. In a few experiments in nephritic rats in which the albumin concentration in tubular fluid rose above 1 mg/ml, albumin absorption rates were significantly higher than would be allowed by the low-capacity system for albumin absorption.[40,44] In these experiments, however, tubular lumens were dilated and it could not be excluded that the higher absorption rates were caused by greater contact time or other tubular function abnormality rather than by the presence of a high-absorptive-capacity system. In the present experiments, high concentrations of albumin did not affect tubular diameter or fluid reabsorption. Consequently, it is likely that the high-absorptive-capacity system is a normal feature of the transport mechanism for albumin absorption by tubular cells.

The exact mechanism(s) for the dual kinetics of albumin absorption are not entirely clear. It is possible that the luminal membrane or the endocytic sites have two or more binding sites with different affinity for albumin. It also cannot be completely ruled out that high albumin concentrations stimulate the rate of endocytic vesicle formation. This possibility is, however, unlikely, since we demonstrated that inulin uptake (a marker of fluid endocytosis and consequently of the rate of formation of endocytic vesicles) is not increased by the presence of high albumin concentrations in the tubular fluid.[3]

We proposed a hypothetical qualitative model that could account for the dual kinetics of albumin uptake.[3] This model is schematically depicted in Fig. 7. Both systems use the endocytic pathway. The low-capacity system (panel A, Fig. 7) is via adsorptive endocytosis, i.e., binding of albumin to luminal sites before the incorporation into the endocytic vesicles. Since albumin is a relatively large anionic protein, it is not surprising that the number of sites is functionally limited, leading to early saturation of this transport system. The high-capacity system (panel B, Fig. 7) may be via the bulk incorporation of albumin aggregates into endocytic vesicles. The formation of albumin aggregates near the endocytic sites at the bottom of the microvilli is favored by the rapid removal of fluid via active Na reabsorption in a relatively narrow space. Naturally, this system would only play an important role at higher luminal fluid albumin concentrations. The high-capacity system would saturate when further access of the albumin molecules to the endocytic sites at the bottom of the microvilli would be limited by electrical and geometric constraints.[28] If the above model is correct, it can be predicted that tubular absorption of albumin, particularly at high filtrate concentrations of this protein, is sensitive to variations in luminal flow rates and fluid reabsorption. It should be pointed out that the presence of a low- and a high-capacity system may not be unique to albumin since, based on clearance experiments in the rabbit, Nomiyama and Foulkes[53] suggested that the absorption of another anionic protein, cadmium-metallothionein, is also characterized by the presence of a dual kinetics of absorption.

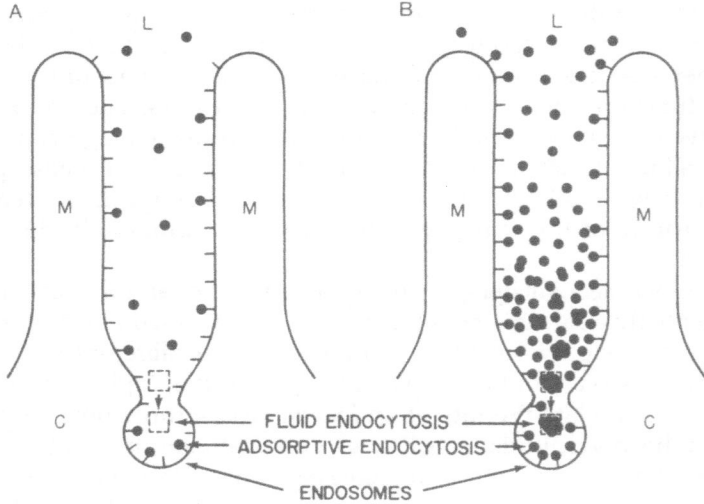

Figure 7. Diagrammatic representation of hypothetical qualitative model to explain the dual kinetics of albumin absorption by isolated perfused proximal tubules of the rabbit. The luminal membrane of proximal convoluted tubules is represented with the tubular lumen (L), microvilli (M), endosomes, and the cell interior (C). Albumin molecules are depicted as filled circles, binding sites by bars, and bulk incorporation into endosomes (fluid endocytosis) by the squares with the arrows. Albumin may be absorbed by two distinct processes. A: Binding of albumin to a finite number of sites with subsequent incorporation into the endosomes (adsorptive endocytosis). This mechanism may be responsible for the low-capacity system that operates at near physiological ranges of tubular fluid albumin concentrations. B: Aggregation of albumin molecules near the base of the microvili with subsequent bulk incorporation of the aggregate in the endocytic vesicle. This mechanism may be responsible for the high-capacity system of albumin absorption and may operate at abnormally high tubular fluid concentrations of albumin. See text. (From Park and Maack[3] with permission.)

Pathophysiological Significance: Albuminuria, Protein Absorption Droplets, and Increased Renal Catabolic Rates of Albumin

Although many aspects of the tubular absorption and catabolism of albumin remain to be elucidated, the data obtained to date already permit a better understanding of the phenomenon of albuminuria and particularly of the relationship among albuminuria, protein absorption droplets, and increased renal catabolic rates of albumin. Increased filtered loads of albumin in glomerular diseases may lead to albuminuria long before the tubular absorption of this protein is saturated. This is because of the relatively low affinity of the absorption process, which entails that at loads below the maximal absorptive capacity, there will be a proportionality between filtered loads and urinary excretion rates of albumin. In view of the presence of a high-absorptive-capacity system, tubular absorption of albumin will continue to increase as filtered loads rise, even in the presence of significant albuminuria. Consequently, in severe glomerular disease, albuminuria may be accompanied by an increase in the renal catabolism of albumin[54] and possibly by the deposition of protein absorption droplets within renal tubular cells.[4,5] These phenomena would be difficult to explain if albumin absorption saturated at near normal filtered loads.

Deposition of protein absorption droplets and increased renal catabolic rates of albumin may not be related, however, to albuminuria in a simple manner. Indeed, in view of the characteristics of the high-capacity absorptive system (see model in Fig. 7 and text above), the degree of tubular absorption of albumin at high luminal concentrations of this protein may be particularly sensitive to tubular flow rates and fluid reabsorption. Both parameters may be altered in renal diseases, affecting the degree of tubular absorption of albumin. Furthermore, as shown for low-molecular-weight proteins, renal cell catabolism of absorbed albumin may depend not solely on the nature of the protein and its rate of tubular absorption but also on the maintenance of an adequate low intralysosomal pH. A high intralysosomal pH, which impairs protein hydrolysis,[2] may occur if lysosomal membrane permeability to protons is increased and/or if the energy supply to the lysosomal membrane proton pump is deficient. These conditions may be present if the glomerular disease is accompanied by tubular cell damage. In view of the above, there need not be a direct correlation between the degree of albuminuria and the increase in renal catabolic rates of albumin or the deposition of protein absorption droplets within the renal cells. In any event, deposition of absorption droplets and increased renal catabolic rates of albumin may have important pathophysiological significance in humans. The former may lead to tubular damage and contribute to the deterioration of renal function in glomerular diseases. An increase in renal catabolic rates of albumin may contribute to the accelerated plasma turnover of this protein and consequently to the hypoalbuminemia of the nephrotic syndrome.

ACKNOWLEDGMENT. Studies from our laboratory described in this chapter were supported by the National Institutes of Health Research Grant AM-14241. Dr. Park was supported by a National Institutes of Health postdoctoral fellowship 5T32 AM-07152 and Dr. Camargo by a fellowship from the Conselho Nacional de Desenvolvimento de Pesquisas Cientificas e Tecnologicas from Brazil.

REFERENCES

1. Maack T, Johnson V, Kau ST, et al: Renal filtration, transport and metabolism of low molecular weight proteins: A review. *Kidney Int* 16:251–270, 1979
2. Maack T, Camargo MJF, Park HC: Renal filtration, transport and metabolism of proteins, in Seldin DW, Giebisch G (eds): *The Kidney: Physiology and Pathophysiology*. New York, Raven Press, 1985
3. Park HC, Maack T: Albumin absorption and catabolism by isolated perfused proximal convoluted tubules of the rabbit. *J Clin Invest* 73:767–777, 1984
4. Oliver J, MacDowell M, Lee YC: Cellular mechanism of protein metabolism in the nephron. I. The structural aspects of proteinuria; tubular absorption, droplet formation, and the disposal of proteins. *J Exp Med* 99:589–604, 1954
5. Oliver J: Transport of macromolecules. Discussion, in Metcoff J (ed): *Proceedings of the 8th Annual Conference on the Nephrotic Syndrome*. New York, New York Academy of Science 1956, pp 1–14
6. Straus W: Segregation of intravenously injected protein by ''droplets'' of cells of rat kidney. *J Biophys Biochem Cytol* 3:1037–1043, 1957
7. Straus W: Occurrence of phagosomes and phago-lysosomes on different nephron segments in relation to the reabsorption, transport, digestion, and extrusion of intravenously injected horseradish peroxidase. *J Cell Biol* 21:295–308, 1964
8. Straus W: Cytochemical observations on the relationship between lysosomes and phagosomes in kidney and liver by combined staining for acid phosphatase and intravenously injected horseradish peroxidase. *J Cell Biol* 20:497–507, 1964
9. Miller F, Palade GE: Lytic activities in renal protein absorption droplets. An electron microscopical cytochemical study. *J Cell Biol* 23:519–552, 1964
10. Maunsbach AB: Absorption of ^{125}I-homologous albumin by rat kidney proximal tubular cells. *J Ultrastruct Res* 15: 197–241, 1966
11. Maack T: Changes in the activity of acid hydrolases during renal reabsorption of lysozyme. *J Cell Biol* 35:268–273, 1967
12. Maack T, Mackensie DDS, Kinter WB: Intracellular pathways of renal absorption of lysozyme. *Am J Physiol* 221:1609–1616, 1971
13. Bourdeau JE, Carone FA, Ganote CE: Serum albumin uptake in isolated perfused renal tubules: Quantitative electron microscope autoradiographic studies in three anatomical segments of the rabbit nephron. *J Cell Biol* 54:382–398, 1972
14. Maack T, Sherman RI: Proteinuria: A combined clinical and basic science seminar. *Am J Med* 56:71–81, 1974
15. Johnson V, Maack T: Renal extraction, filtration, absorption, and catabolism of growth hormone. *Am J Physiol* 233:F189–F196, 1977
16. Maack T: Renal handling of low molecular weight proteins. *Am J Med* 56:57–64, 1975
17. Kau ST, Maack T: Transport and catabolism of parathyroid hormone in isolated rat kidney. *Am J Physiol* 233:F445–F454, 1977
18. Maack T, Sigulem D: Renal handling of lysozyme, in Osserman EF (ed): *Lysozyme*. New York, Academic Press, 1974, pp 321–333
19. Rabinovitch M, Dohi SR: Increase in serum ribonuclease activity after bilateral nephrectomy. *Am J Physiol* 187:525–528, 1956
20. Wochner RD, Strober W, Waldmann TA: The role of the kidney in the catabolism of Bence Jones proteins and immunoglobulin fragments. *J Exp Med* 126:207–220, 1967
21. Hayslett JP, Perrilie PE, Finch SC: Urinary muramidase and renal disease. *N Engl J Med* 279:506–512, 1968

22. Royce PC: Characterization of renal-dependent rat serum protein. *Am J Physiol* 215:1429–1434, 1968
23. Martin TJ, Mellick RA, DeLuise M: The effect of nephrectomy on the metabolism of labelled parathyroid hormone. *Clin Sci* 37:137–142, 1969
24. Keeler R: The effect of bilateral nephrectomy on the production and distribution of muramidase (lysozyme) in the rat. *Can J Physiol Pharmacol* 48:131–138, 1970
25. Wallace ALC, Stacy BD: Disappearance rate of ^{125}I-labelled rat growth hormone in nephrectomized and sham operated rats. *Horm Metab Res* 7:135–138, 1975
26. Katz AI, Rubenstein AH: Metabolism of proinsulin, insulin and C-peptide in the rat. *J Clin Invest* 52:1113–1121, 1973
27. Rabkin R, Kitabachi AE: Factors influencing the handling of insulin by the isolated rat kidney. *J Clin Invest* 62:169–175, 1978
28. Sumpio BE, Maack T: Kinetics, competition and selectivity of tubular absorption of proteins. *Am J Physiol* 243:F379–F392, 1982
29. Muggia FM, Heinemann HO, Farhangi M, et al: Lysozymuria and renal tubular disfuction in monocytic and myelomonocytic leukemia. *Am J Med* 47:351–365, 1969
30. Koss MN, Pirani CL, Osserman EF: Experimental Bence Jones cast nephropathy. *Lab Invest* 34: 579–591, 1976
31. Cojocel CM, Franzen-Sieveking M, Beckman G, et al: Inhibition of renal accumulation of lysozyme (basic low molecular weight protein) by basic proteins and other basic substances. *Pfluegers Arch* 390:211–215, 1981
32. Carone FA, Peterson DR: Hydrolysis and transport of small peptides by the proximal tubule. *Am J Physiol* 238:F151–F158, 1980
33. Hruska KA, Martin K, Mendes A, et al: Degradation of parathyroid hormone and fragment production by the isolated perfused dog kidney. *J Clin Invest* 60:501–510, 1977
34. Sumpio BE: *Tubular Absorption and Catabolism of Low Molecular Weight Proteins.* Thesis, New York, Cornell University, 1981
35. Cortney MA, Sawin LL, Weiss DD: Renal tubular protein absorption in the rat. *J Clin Invest* 49:1–4, 1970
36. Dirks JH, Clapp JR, Berliner RW: The protein concentration in the proximal tubule of the dog. *J Clin Invest* 45:916–921, 1964
37. Leber PD, Marsh DJ: Micropuncture study of concentration and fate of albumin in rat nephron. *Am J Physiol* 219:358–363, 1970
38. Oken DE, Flamenbaum W: Micropuncture studies of proximal tubule albumin concentrations in normal and nephrotic rats. *J Clin Invest* 50:1498–1505, 1971
39. Oken DE, Cotes SC, Mende CW: Micropuncture study of tubular transport of albumin in rats with aminonucleoside nephrosis. *Kidney Int* 1:3–11, 1972
40. Lewy JE, Pesce AJ: Micropuncture study of albumin transfer in aminonucleoside nephrosis in the rat. *Pediatr Res* 7:553–559, 1973
41. Eisenbach GM, Van Liew JB, Boylan JW: Effects of angiotensin on filtration of protein in the rat kidney: A micropuncture study. *Kidney Int* 8:80–87, 1975
42. Von Bayer H, Van Liew JB, Klassen J, et al: Filtration of protein in anti-glomerular basement membrane nephritic rat: A micropuncture study. *Kidney Int* 10:425–437, 1976
43. Landwehr DM, Carvalho JS, Oken DE: Micropuncture studies of the filtration and absorption of albumin by nephrotic rats. *Kidney Int* 11:9–17, 1977
44. Galaske RG, Baldamus CA, Stolte H: Plasma protein handling in the rat kidney. Micropuncture experiments in the acute phase of anti-GBM-nephritis. *Pfluegers Arch* 375:269–277, 1978
45. Burg MB, Orloff J: Control of fluid absorption in the renal proximal tubule. *J Clin Invest* 47:2016–2024, 1968

46. Friedman PA, Figueiredo JF, Maack T, et al: Sodium–calcium interactions in the renal proximal convoluted tubule of the rabbit. *Am J Physiol* 240:F558–F568, 1981
47. Tack FF, Dean J, Eliat PE, et al: Tritium labelling of proteins to high specific radioactivity by reductive methylation. *J Biol Chem* 285:8842–8847, 1980
48. Park CH, Maack T: Albumin (ALB) absorption and metabolism by proximal convoluted tubules of the rabbit: Dissociation from fluid reabsorption by chloroquine (CQ). *Fed Proc* 42:480, 1983
49. Just M, Haberman E: The renal handling of polybasic drugs: In vitro studies with brush border and lysosomal preparations. *Naunyn-Schmiedebergs Arch Pharmacol* 300:67–76, 1977
50. Christensen EI, Carone FA, Rennke HG: Effect of molecular charge on endocytic uptake of ferritin in renal proximal tubule cells. *Lab Invest* 44:351–358, 1981
51. Hoare D, Koshland D: A method for the quantitative modification and estimation of carxylic acid groups in proteins. *J Biol Chem* 242:2447–2453, 1967
52. Bohrer MP, Baylis C, Humes HD, et al: Permselectivity of the glomerular capillary wall: Facilitated filtration of circulating polycations. *J Clin Invest* 61:72–78, 1978
53. Nomiyama K, Foulkes EC: Reabsorption of filtered cadmium-metallothionein in the rabbit kidney. *Proc Soc Exp Biol Med* 156:97–99, 1977
54. Katz J, Bonoris G, Sellers AL: Albumin metabolism in aminonucleoside nephrotic rats. *J Lab Clin Med* 62:910–934, 1963

4

Tubular Proteinuria
Clinical Implications*

JOHN F. MAHER

INTRODUCTION

Proteinuria was recognized and associated with renal disease almost two centuries ago by Dekkers and by Cotugno.[1] As recently as 1950, however, the proteinuria of renal disease was considered to result from the same mechanisms for all abnormalities.[2,3] Although restricted passage of protein through glomerular capillaries was identified, it was also appreciated that the limited sensitivity of the protein assay used in the micropuncture studies of Walker, Bott, Oliver, and MacDowell[4] could not detect proteinuria below 300 mg/liter. Therefore, it was judged that as much as 50 g of protein could be filtered and reabsorbed daily by normal tubules. Although many investigators focused exclusively on the glomerular barrier, Addis,[5] Oliver,[6] and Dock[7] favored significant protein reabsorption because of the detection of protein markers in absorption droplets in tubular epithelial cells and the occurrence of proteinuria when tubular activity is inhibited while filtration persists. Nevertheless, attention was directed almost exclusively toward the overt and often disabling proteinuria of glomerular origin until a peculiar proteinuria of low molecular weight was identified in patients with cadmium intoxication by Friberg[8] and until the proteinuria of tubular disorders was described by Butler and Flynn.[9]

---

*The opinions and assertions contained herein are those of the author and are not to be construed as official or as representing those of the Uniformed Services University of the Health Sciences or the Department of Defense.

JOHN F. MAHER • Department of Medicine, Nephrology Division, Uniformed Services University of the Health Sciences School of Medicine, Bethesda, Maryland 20817.

It is now apparent that there are several mechanism for the appearance of protein in the urine depending on the causative abnormality. Boylan[10] categorizes proteinuria into five types as listed in Table I. Whereas the albumin concentration in glomerular filtrate is normally less than 0.1% of the plasma concentration, the low-molecular-weight proteins are not so restricted.[11,12] At an average molecular mass of about 20,000 daltons, the filtrate concentration of small proteins may exceed half that of plasma. Despite a much lower plasma concentration, the filtered load of low-molecular-weight proteins would thus be somewhat higher than that of albumin, i.e., above 500 mg daily. About 95% of filtered protein is reabsorbed normally, so urinary excretion is approximately 25 mg of albumin daily and slightly more of low-molecular-weight protein. To this is added a small amount of secreted protein, predominantly Tamm Horsfall uromucoid. Total urinary protein is normally less than 100 mg daily.

The low-molecular-weight proteins have low sedimentation coefficients and electrophoretic mobility mainly in the α_2- and β-globulin regions. Their concentrations in glomerular filtrate relate directly to their plasma concentrations and indirectly to their molecular dimensions. Below 25 Å, the filtrate concentration is 95% or more of the plasma concentration. The protein species listed in Table II are those that permeate the glomerulus readily, appearing in the urine when reabsorption is impaired, and include enzymes, polypeptide hormones, immunoglobulin fragments, and other small proteins.[11-13]

TUBULAR TRANSPORT OF PROTEIN

Renal tubular reabsorption occurs by pinocytosis. The initial event is binding of free amino or guanidino groups of the protein to negatively charged sites on the cell.[14] This is followed by rapid ingress into the tubular cell from the lumen via brush border apical vesicles, which form

Table I. Proteinuria

Type	Mechanism	Example of urinary protein
Glomerular	↑Permeability	Albumin
Tubular	↓Reabsorption	β_2-Microglobulin
Overflow	↑Plasma concentration	Light chains
Secretory	Inflammation	IgA
Histuria	Tissue necrosis	Myoglobin

Table II. Protein Species in Tubular Proteinuria

30–50 protein species
Enzymes
  Amylase, lysozyme, ribonuclease
Polypeptide hormones
  Calcitonin, FSH, LH, glucagon, growth hormone, insulin, PTH, prolactin
Polyclonal immunoglobulin fragments; x and λ light chains (monomers and dimers)
Fibrin and fibrin degradation products
Retinol binding protein, α_2-microglobulin β_2-microglobulin, post-γ proteins

---

phagosomes that migrate away from the luminal border and fuse with lysosomes, where hydrolytic proteases catabolize the proteins over the course of minutes to days.[11,12,15] Eventually, the catabolized fragments are discharged on the antiluminal surface. Only a small fraction of reabsorbed protein escapes catabolism and is returned to the circulation intact. The impermeability of the basal surface of the tubule to protein is consistent with the long residual time in the cell and the absence of movement of protein from peritubular capillaries into the cell.

Characteristics of tubular protein reabsorption are as follows. It occurs in the proximal tubule and is nonselective and competitive.[11,15,16] Accordingly, when reabsorption is blocked, there is no change in the excretory ratio of x and λ light chains or of the monomers and dimers of these immunoglobulin fragments.[17] When overflow proteinuria occurs because of excessive production of light chains or of lysozyme, all small proteins should appear in the urine in increased quantities. Similarly, when increased glomerular permeability raises the filtered load of albumin, the reabsorption of small proteins is competitively inhibited, and their excretion rate increases about fivefold. In contrast, tubular damage can increase excretion of these proteins about 50-fold.[17] Experimentally, a high casein intake also increases the fractional excretion of low-molecular-weight proteins.[18] Hence, the reabsorptive process is saturable. The reabsorptive process is of high capacity and low affinity. Although saturable, absolute reabsorption may increase as fractional reabsorption decreases. Protein reabsorption by the tubule can be selectively inhibited by lysine or other cationic substances that interfere with the negative charge on the brush border. The reabsorptive process requires expenditure of energy. Accordingly, it is blocked by cyanide, maleate, or iodoacetate.

There is no evidence that the low-molecular-weight proteins are secreted. They are not eliminated by the non-filtering kidney. Renal arterial occlusion or nephrectomy abolishes elimination of these proteins, whereas total urinary obstruction does not. Thus, these solutes are eliminated by glomerular filtration. Since they do not appear normally in urine except in minute quantities, they are virtually completely reabsorbed. Proximal tubular injury results in low molecular weight proteinuria. Hence, the elimination process also conserves nitrogen. Unlike sodium and many other solutes, impaired proximal reabsorption is not compensated by a more distal mechanism and the reabsorptive process is not so affected by hemodynamic, hormonal and dietary influences. In the absence of increased plasma levels, low molecular weight proteinuria is a good marker, therefore, of proximal tubular injury.

CLINICAL CORRELATIONS

Table III lists the diseases that cause tubular proteinuria.[9,11,19-22] Detection of tubular proteinuria can thus be clinically useful in the diagnosis of a variety of renal lesions and in monitoring specific disease processes.

Monitoring of industrial exposure to such toxins as cadmium can be facilitated by measurement of specific urinary proteins, thereby increasing safety. Similarly, early evidence of tubular dysfunction from such drugs as gentamicin can be detected by tubular proteinuria. Such changes imply impaired function and not necessarily tubular injury; however, impending renal failure may be predicted more accurately however, by detecting increased secretory proteinuria such as Tamm Horsfall (urinary casts) or N-acetylglucosaminidase.[23,24] Tubular proteinuria does not occur with lower urinary tract infection but is detected with a high frequency when infection involves the kidney.[25] A variety of renal diseases that cause tubular proteinuria can be complicated by urinary tract infection, so diagnostic accuracy is limited. Preexisting tubular proteinuria renders the test much less useful for distinguishing the site of infection. On the other hand, detection of tubular proteinuria is a useful means of distinguishing preexisting renal disease mimicking toxemia from true preeclampsia.[26] The occurrence of tubular proteinuria in patients with vesicoureteral reflux should be considered an indicator of renal injury. Moreover, although proteinuria may complicate renal ischemia associated with hemodynamic changes in glomeruli, the occurrence of tubular proteinuria should suggest renal injury rather than a physiological response.

When membranous glomerulonephritis involves antecedent renal tubular injury followed by an immunologic reaction to renal tubular epithelial antigens, this problem can be distinguished from other causes of the nephrotic syndrome by the presence of tubular proteinuria.

Table III. Causes of Tubular Proteinuria

Congenital
  Fanconi syndrome, occulocerebrorenal dystrophy, renal tubular acidosis, Bartter's syndrome, familial asymptomatic tubular proteinuria
Systemic disease
  Hereditary
    Wilson's disease, galactosemia, glycogen storage disease, cystinosis oxalosis
  Acquired
    sarcoidosis, multiple myeloma, Balkan nephropathy, lupus erythematosus
Drugs
  Acute hypersensitivity interstitial nephritis (methicillin), laxative abuse, aminoglycoside toxicity, analgesic nephropathy
Heavy metals and poisons
  Cd, Pb, As, Hg, ethylene glycol, CCl_4
Acute renal disease
  Tubular necrosis, transplant rejection
Infection
  Pyelonephritis
Miscellaneous
  Hypercalcemia, hyperparathyroidism, nephronophthisis, vesicoureteral reflux, obstructive uropathy

Hardwicke[27] has correlated the presence of tubular proteinuria with the tubulointerstitial abnormalities associated with renal failure and suggests that when such proteinuria develops in nephrotic children the prognosis is worse, and more vigorous treatment should be considered. Finally, because tubular reabsorption can be reversibly blocked, assessment of the filtered load of small proteins can be used to judge the mass of a variety of tumors.[27] Multiple myeloma is such an example. This technique could be also applied to the evaluation of various endocrine adenomas and to assess the protein elimination rate in nephrotic syndrome.

There are several limitations and pitfalls in the clinical determination of tubular proteinuria. Any increase in production rate of a low-molecular-weight protein raises the plasma concentration and therefore the filtered load, leading to overflow proteinuria as reabsorption is saturated. Increased glomerular permeability will also raise the filtered load of proteins including any small proteins that are partially sieved. Moreover, as low-molecular-weight proteins are retained with renal failure, the consequent high plasma level results in an increased filtered load per nephron.[28] Each of these circumstances will cause proteinuria by competitive inhibition of tubular reabsorption rather than by specific failure of the tubule. The quantitative increase should be less than that induced by tubular disease, but it could require a reversible inhibition, e.g., by lysine, to demonstrate that appreciable reabsorption is occurring.

Hyperparathyroidism or hypercalcemia can complicate renal disease, and each of these can inhibit proximal tubular function inducing proteinuria.[21,29] Moreover, the exposure to a variety of drugs can transiently inhibit protein reabsorption without inducing tubular damage.[30] Accordingly, tubular proteinuria does not necessarily indicate that the primary abnormality causing renal disease resides in the tubule.

β_2-Microglobulin is the low-molecular-weight protein most frequently measured to screen for tubular proteinuria because of the simplicity of the radioimmunoassay. It is a 100-amino-acid chain with a single disulfide bridge and a molecular mass of 11,600 daltons. The production of β_2-microglobulin, which is linked to the histocompatibility antigens, is relatively stable. In an acid urine, however, the molecule deteriorates. Retinol binding protein is a more reliable indicator of tubular proteinuria when urinary pH is below 6.0.[31] Furthermore, the occurrence of β_2-microglobulinuria in some patients with glomerular diseases makes it a less reliable discriminator between tubulointerstitial and glomerular diseases than lysozyme is.[32] Lysozyme, on the other hand, is produced by monocytes, and urinary excretion increases in patients with leukemia.[33] Accordingly, measurement of the excretion rate of a single protein may give misleading results, but even increased excretion of many low-molecular-weight proteins can occur for reasons other than tubular injury, some of which are inconsequential.

There is no specific pattern of tubular proteinuria that would distinguish any particular renal tubular lesion from all others. Detection of tubular proteinuria identifies impaired proximal tubular function but does not discriminate among the causes.[34,35] The diagnosis of a specific renal tubular disease ordinarily depends on identification of pertinent historical information or by recognition of associated systemic abnormalities. Occasionally, a characteristic morphological change can be seen by imaging techniques or histological study of renal biopsy specimens, but these may show only nonspecific changes. Nevertheless, tubular proteinuria is a manifestation that segregates a group of renal diseases from others implicating proximal tubular dysfunction, just as nephrotic syndrome implies glomerular dysfunction, separating its causes from many other entities that afflict the kidney.

Once tubular proteinuria is identified, clinical evaluation requires numerous considerations. Medical history of pertinent familial abnormalities, bone pain, renal transplant, arthritis, and exposure to drugs and toxins should be sought. The latter includes the many causes of acute interstitial nephritis, drugs that cause potassium depletion, the aminoglycosides, halogenated hydrocarbons, heavy metals, and mixed analgesics. This often requires more than simple questioning and should include inquiry about the patient's occupation, hobbies, and lifestyle.

Loin pain, fever, and dysuria suggest pyelonephritis. Bone pain, weakness, and recurrent infections may indicate myeloma. Clinical symptoms of lupus erythematosus should also be sought.

Frequently, the physical examination adds little to diagnostic information, but it is important to register the blood pressure, search diligently for corneal opacification, Kayser–Fleischer rings, arthritis, dermatitis, and other signs of systemic lupus, hepatomegaly, stigmata of cirrhosis, and renal enlargement.

Laboratory evidence of hypercalcemia, hypokalemia, light-chain immunoglobulinemia, galactosemia, hyperparathyroidism, anti-DNA antibodies, hemolytic anemia, or hypoceruloplasminemia can focus the diagnostic possibilities. Hyperuricemia frequently accompanies renal disease, but associated clinical gout is rare and suggests urate retention as a result of lead nephropathy. Hypouricemia, an unusual finding, suggests Fanconi syndrome and such abnormalities as cadmium intoxication and Wilson's disease. Phosphaturia, glycosuria, aminoaciduria, and proximal renal tubular acidosis imply the diffuse proximal tubular transport abnormalities of Fanconi syndrome. Eosinophiluria suggests hypersensitivity interstitial nephritis, whereas detection of N-acetyl-*para*-aminophenol in the urine implies analgesic use. Sterile pyuria is often seen with analgesic nephropathy, whereas bacteriuria may suggest pyelonephritis.

Renal imaging techniques can confirm the diagnosis of urinary tract obstruction, papillary necrosis, vesicoureteral reflux, and nephronophthisis.

Renal biopsy may be required to establish the diagnosis of transplant rejection, sarcoid granulomatous nephritis, tubular necrosis, acute or chronic interstitial nephritis, myeloma kidney, nephrocalcinosis, or lupus nephritis. Histochemical demonstration of copper, lead, gold, calcium, cystine, oxalate, or glycogen may be required in addition to the usual immunofluorescent and electron microscopic studies of the tissue.

Of the various causes of tubular proteinuria, some are preventable, and others are reversible, but many can only be managed supportively at this time. It is important to distinguish the specific renal disease in order to provide rational treatment. Further understanding of the mechanisms of injury provides hope for improved therapy for the future.

REFERENCES

1. Major RH: *Classic Descriptions of Disease*, ed 3. Springfield, IL, Charles C Thomas, 1945, p 677
2. Smith HW: *The Kidney: Structure and Function in Health and Disease*. New York, Oxford University Press, 1951, p 1049

3. Fishberg AM: *Hypertension and Nephritis*, ed 5. Philadelphia, Lea & Febiger, 1954, p 986
4. Walker AM, Bott PA, Oliver J, et al: The collection and analysis of fluid from single nephrons of the mammalian kidney. *Am J Physiol* 134:580–595, 1941
5. Addis T: Proteinuria. *Trans Assoc Am Physicians* 57:106–108, 1942
6. Oliver J: The structure of the metabolic process in the nephron. *J Mt Sinai Hosp* 15:175–222, 1948
7. Dock W: Proteinuria and the associated renal changes. *N Engl J Med* 227:633–636, 1942
8. Friberg L: Health hazards in the manufacture of alkaline accumulators with special reference to chronic cadmium poisoning. *Acta Med Scand [Suppl]* 240:1–124, 1950
9. Butler EA, Flynn FV: The proteinuria of renal tubular disorders. *Lancet* 2:978–980, 1958
10. Boylan JW: Introduction. *Kidney Int* 16:247–250, 1979
11. Hall CL, Hardwicke J: Low molecular weight proteinuria. *Annu Rev Med* 30:199–211, 1979
12. Maack T, Johnson V, Kau ST, et al: Renal filtration, transport and metabolism of low-molecular-weight proteins: A review. *Kidney Int* 16:251–270, 1979
13. Edwards JJ, Tollaksen SL, Anderson NG: Proteins of human urine. III. Identification and two-dimensional electrophoretic map positions of some major urinary proteins. *Clin Chem* 28:941–948, 1982
14. Mogensen CE, Sølling K: Studies on renal tubular protein reabsorption: Partial and near complete inhibition by certain amino acids. *Scand J Clin Lab Invest* 37:477–486, 1977
15. Bordeau JE, Carone FA: Protein handling by the renal tubule. *Nephron* 13:22–34, 1974
16. Baumann K, Cojocel C: Microperfusion and clearance studies on renal protein reabsorption. *Contrib Nephrol* 24:8–17, 1981
17. Sølling K: Light chain polymerism in normal individuals with severe proteinuria and in normals with inhibited tubular protein reabsorption by lysine. *Scand J Clin Lab Invest* 40:129–134, 1980
18. Neuhaus OW, Flory W, Biswas N, et al: Urinary excretion of $\alpha_2\mu$-globulin and albumin by adult male rats following treatment with nephrotoxic agents. *Nephron* 28:133–140, 1981
19. Revillard JP, Manuel Y, Francois R, et al: Renal disease associated with tubular proteinuria, in Manuel Y, Revillard JP, Betuel H (eds): *Proteins in Normal and Pathological Urine*. Basel, S Karger, 1970, pp 209–219
20. Killingsworth LM: Clinical applications of protein determinations in biological fluids other than blood. *Clin Chem* 28:1093–1102, 1982
21. Morgan DB: Assessment of renal tubular function and damage and their clinical significance. *Ann Clin Biochem* 19:307–313, 1982
22. Flynn FV, Platt HS: The origin of the proteins excreted in tubular proteinuria. *Clin Chem Acta* 21:377–399, 1968
23. Feig PU, Mitchell PP, Abrutyn E, et al: Aminoglycoside nephrotoxicity; a double-blind prospective randomized study of gentamicin and tobramycin. *J Antimicrob Chemother* 10:217–226, 1982
24. Powell JH, Reidenberg MM: In vitro responses of rat and human kidney lysosomes to aminoglycosides. *Biochem Pharmacol* 31:3447–3453, 1982
25. Mengoli C, Lechi A, Arosio E, et al: Contribution of four markers of tubular proteinuria in detecting upper urinary tract infections. A multivariate analysis. *Nephron* 32:234–238, 1982
26. Weise M, Prüfer D, Jacques G, et al: β_2-Microglobulin and other proteins as parameter for tubular function. *Contrib Nephrol* 24:88–98, 1981
27. Hardwicke J: Proteinuria—the future? *Clin Nephrol* 21:50–53, 1984
28. Harrison JF, Blainey JD: Low molecular weight proteinuria in chronic renal disease. *Clin Sci* 33:381–390, 1967

29. Hey H, Skaarup P, Sølling K, et al: Tubular proteinuria following jejuno-ileal bypass surgery. *Int J Obesity* 5:155-161, 1981
30. Fleming JJ, Cooper EH, Hay AMW, et al: Tubuloproteinuria in cancer chemotherapy. *Rec Clin Lab* 10:135-141, 1980
31. Bernard AM, Moreau D, Lauwerys R: Comparison of retinol-binding protein and β_2-microglobulin determination in urine for the early detection of tubular proteinuria. *Clin Chim Acta* 126:1-7, 1982
32. Zager RA: Urinary protein markers of tubulointerstitial nephritis. *Invest Urol* 18:197-202, 1981
33. Osserman EF, Lawlor DP: Serum and urinary lysozyme (muramidase) in monocytic and monomyelocytic leukemia. *J Exp Med* 124:921-952, 1966
34. Creeth JM, Kekwick RA, Flynn FV, et al: An ultracentrifuge study of urine proteins with particular reference to the proteinuria of tubular disorders. *Clin Chim Acta* 8:406-414, 1963
35. Zager RA: Proteinuria of tubulointerstitial nephritis: Diagnostic considerations. *Contrib Nephrol* 35:180-190, 1983

5

Clinical Significance of Isolated Proteinuria

ROSCOE R. ROBINSON

INTRODUCTION

Diagnostic and prognostic uncertainty often surrounds the qualitative detection of proteinuria in asymptomatic individuals who seem otherwise healthy. Such uncertainty can be most pronounced when proteinuria is modest in amount and unaccompanied by any other clinical or laboratory abnormality. The unsuspected finding of isolated proteinuria on routine urinalysis can give rise to two important questions: (1) does proteinuria reflect the underlying presence of some form of kidney disease, and if so, (2) will the disease eventually cause morbidity or death? Unfortunately, it is not always possible to answer either question with confidence, at least on first examination of an individual patient.

Several factors have contributed to this state of affairs: (1) the long-standing recognition that proteinuria can and does occur in the absence of underlying kidney disease; (2) the equally convincing demonstration that isolated proteinuria may also be accompanied by histological alterations of kidney structure and that some such changes are sufficient to warrant a firm diagnosis of kidney disease[1-13]; (3) the possibility that the incidence of casual proteinuria in young adults may be greater than that of subsequent death from renal failure,[14] suggesting again that kidney disease may not exist in all such patients or that, if it does, it may not always achieve future clinical significance as a cause of mortality; (4) an awareness that conclusions derived from a study of isolated proteinuria in one age or population group may not necessarily apply to another; (5) the historical application of a profuse array of descriptive terms to pro-

ROSCOE R. ROBINSON • Department of Medicine, Vanderbilt University Medical Center, Nashville, Tennessee 37232.

teinuria in apparently healthy individuals, e.g., juvenile, orthostatic, constant, cyclic, persistent, intermittent, isolated, benign, transient, minimal, physiological, or functional. In some instances, the criteria for the use of these terms have not been defined clearly; in others, the criteria may be clear, but they differ from those of others, thereby complicating the comparison of the results of one study with another.

For these reasons, exact definition of the proteinuric population under consideration is of great importance. This discussion focuses on a large population of young adults whose proteinuria is noted first as an "isolated" clinical finding. Isolated proteinuria is often discovered during a routine health examination, perhaps in preparation for entrance into military service, participation in athletics, or application for life insurance or employment. The term "isolated" proteinuria should only apply to patients who are asymptomatic and apparently healthy at the time of initial examination and who exhibit no evidence of systemic disease, impaired kidney function, or abnormalities of the urine sediment. Excretory urography and nuclear or ultrasonographic imaging studies are within normal limits, and there is no antecedent history of kidney or urologic disease. Total urine protein excretion is usually less than 1.0 g per day. Most patients are in the younger age groups at the time of initial diagnosis, but the apparent validity of this statement is undoubtedly influenced by a relative lack of comparable surveys in older populations. Neither the incidence nor prevalence of isolated proteinuria is certain. Estimates of the incidence of proteinuria on routine urinalysis have varied widely among differing populations, ranging from values as low as 0.6% to those as high as 8.8%.[15-18]

CLASSIFICATION OF ISOLATED PROTEINURIA

When qualitative proteinuria is found as an isolated finding, it can be useful to classify it further according to one of two simple clinical schemes (Table I). First, repetitive routine urinalyses without regard to body posture will demonstrate that proteinuria is "persistent," "transient," or "intermittent" in its occurrence; they will also confirm whether proteinuria is isolated and unaccompanied by other abnormalities of the urine sediment. Second, repetitive examination of the relationship between qualitative proteinuria and changes of body posture will determine if the proteinuria is "constant" in both recumbency and the quiet upright ambulatory posture, "fixed and orthostatic" if present consistently in the upright posture only, or "transient and orthostatic" if observed inconstantly during the upright posture alone.[19,20] Multiple urinalyses

Table I. Qualitative Patterns of Proteinuria

I. On repetitive urinalysis without regard to body posture (routine casual urinalysis)
    A. Persistent
    B. Transient or intermittent
II. On repetitive urinalysis with regard to body posture (serial urine collection test)
    A. Constant in recumbent and upright postures
       a. Persistent
       b. Transient or intermittent
    B. Orthostatic
       a. Fixed
       b. Transient or intermittent

---

must be performed at the time of initial examination if these qualitative patterns are to be identified correctly. It must be emphasized that these so-called "types" or "patterns" of proteinuria probably reflect little more than arbitrarily descriptive laboratory designations, and they should not be viewed as specific clinical entities or syndromes. Any of these qualitative patterns may be the consequence of diverse causes and mechanisms. Moreover, all of them may appear in the same patient at different times during a prolonged period of observation. The reproducibility of a given pattern in a single patient has only been established over relatively short periods of observation.

Several studies have dealt with the clinical significance of persistent versus intermittent proteinuria as determined on repetitive and routine urinalysis without regard to body posture. A detailed consideration of the results of such studies is beyond the scope of this discussion. Possible differences between the clinical significance of persistent and intermittent proteinuria are perhaps reflected well by the results of a follow-up evaluation of former university students who were known to have exhibited qualitative proteinuria on entrance into the university in 1925.[14] Forty-one years later, their mortality rate was compared with that of presumably healthy 18-year-olds who had undergone an examination for life insurance in 1925 and whose routine urinalyses were negative for protein. The subsequent mortality rate was significantly higher in patients who had exhibited proteinuria in more than 80% of a repetitive series of initial urinalyses, i.e., those whose proteinuria was relatively persistent during an initial short-term period of evaluation. These findings imply that the long-term outlook is worse when proteinuria is found to be persistent during the period of initial examination.

Another study dealt with a small group of patients with persistent proteinuria as an isolated finding; i.e., it was not accompanied by other clinical or laboratory abnormalities.[1] Renal biopsy specimens from most of these patients were found to exhibit a heterogeneous spectrum of underlying renal morphological alterations. Nevertheless, only a small fraction of these patients developed renal insufficiency, and then only after long periods of follow-up ranging from 8 to 28 years. It was concluded that progression to renal failure was remarkably indolent in patients who first presented with proteinuria as an isolated finding, even in the presence of underlying renal pathology. The additional finding of microscopic hematuria on initial examination was accompanied by a more rapid progression of renal functional impairment in patients who were otherwise similar.

One of three, possibly four, qualitative patterns may emerge in an individual patient when the appearance of proteinuria is related to changes of body posture (Table II). For many years we have used a simple serial urine collection test to relate the qualitative appearance of proteinuria to changes of body posture.[19,20] When the test is conducted during moderate antidiuresis, results are reproducible in the same patient over short periods of time. On the morning after overnight fluid deprivation, two or more urine samples are collected consecutively during each of two sequentially assumed body postures: recumbency and quiet upright ambulation. Artificial upright lordosis is not induced. A qualitative test for protein (10% sulfosalicylic acid) and a measurement of urine osmolality are performed on each urine sample.

Constant proteinuria (present in both recumbency and the quiet, upright posture; Table II) occurs in approximately 5% to 10% of young men whose proteinuria is first detected on routine urinalysis in which posture is not controlled.[20] It is usually found to be persistent during the repetitive performance of serial urine collection tests; transient or intermittent occurrence is a theoretical possibility, but it has thus far been unreported. Fixed and reproducible orthostatic proteinuria (present consistently on repetitive examination in the upright posture only) occurs in approximately 15% to 20% of young men whose proteinuria is detected initially on casual urinalysis.[20] Transient orthostatic proteinuria (present inconstantly during the upright posture alone) is said by King to be the most common of these posturally defined patterns, perhaps occurring in 70% to 75% of young men in whom isolated proteinuria is first detected on routine urinalysis.[20] Unfortunately, transient orthostatic proteinuria has been studied far less thoroughly than has either fixed orthostatic proteinuria or constant proteinuria. Approximate incidence figures for these types of proteinuria are available only for young men; similar figures are not available for women or other age groups.

Quantitative measurements of total protein excretion have been carried out in patients with clear evidence of constant proteinuria or fixed

Table II. Qualitative Patterns of Isolated Proteinuria

Type	Qualitative Proteinuria				Urine sed.	Kidney function	Systemic disease	Frequency[a]	Definite renal pathology
	supine		upright						
	Day 1	2	Day 1	2					
Constant	+	+	+	+	Neg	Nl	No	5-10%	40-70%
Fixed orthostatic	0	0	+	+	Neg	Nl	No	15-20%	10%
Transient orthostatic	0	0	0	0	Neg	Nl	No	70-80%	Unknown; very low

[a]Among patients with qualitative proteinuria on initial routine urinalysis.

orthostatic proteinuria. Total protein excretion is often higher even during recumbency in patients with fixed orthostatic proteinuria than in healthy patients whose urine is protein-negative in the recumbent and upright postures,[21,22] but the amount of excreted protein is not sufficiently high to permit detection with the usual qualitative tests. The significance of this finding has not been established, nor is its occurrence known to be universal in patients whose qualitative pattern of orthostatic proteinuria is other than that termed fixed and reproducible. Indeed, quantitative protein excretion during recumbency may well be within normal limits in patients with transient orthostatic proteinuria.[23]

CONSTANT PROTEINURIA

For many years, constant proteinuria during both recumbency and the upright posture has been regarded as *prima facie* evidence of underlying kidney disease. Definite morphological evidence of diverse forms of disease has been found on renal biopsy in many instances. It is likely that most of these patients would be found to exhibit persistent proteinuria on repetitive routine urinalysis without postural control. In view of the marked diversity of the underlying renal pathology, it is illogical to expect that all such patients will exhibit an identical clinical course. Nevertheless, the clinical course is apt to be remarkably indolent in the absence of other indicators of active disease such as microscopic hematuria. Few long-term follow-up studies of patients with constant proteinuria have been performed, but the results of one study demonstrated that approximately 80% of such patients still exhibited constant proteinuria after an average 6-year period. Of these, the majority had developed an abnormal urine sediment, and almost 50% had developed mild hypertension, but very few had developed renal insufficiency.[12,13]

ORTHOSTATIC PROTEINURIA

In contrast to constant proteinuria, orthostatic proteinuria has long been regarded as a benign and transient condition not associated with underlying kidney disease.[24-26] This concept of the disorder may well be true in many patients, especially in children and adolescents. Other observations, however, have suggested that orthostatic proteinuria may be a reflection of incipient kidney disease, at least in some patients.[13,27] Light-microscopic studies of kidney biopsy specimens from young men with fixed orthostatic proteinuria revealed that 8% had unequivocal evidence of renal disease, 45% had subtle but definite alterations of glomerular structure (segmental or generalized capillary wall thickening without alterations of the basement membrane, or focal and segmental hypercellularity), and 47% exhibited a histological pattern that appeared normal.[9] A limited number of electron-microscopic observations have confirmed a subtle form of segmental and focal glomerular alterations,[10,28] and immunohistological studies have shown that both immunoglobulin and complement are localized within such foci.[29] Recent histological observations in patients with intermittent orthostatic proteinuria demonstrate minimal changes without immunoprotein on immunofluorescence microscopy, but only a small number of such patients have been studied.[11]

The mechanism by which assumption of the quiet upright posture effects increased protein excretion is uncertain. Regardless of the exact nature of the glomerular changes just described, their existence provides one possible explanation for the proteinuria, that is, an underlying capillary wall alteration or defect that might lead to an increased transglomerular passage of plasma proteins. By itself, however, the existence of an altered capillary wall does not explain abnormal protein excretion occurring only during quiet upright ambulation.[21] The results of earlier studies suggested that any one of the several renal hemodynamic adjustments to standing might serve as the primary cause of orthostatic proteinuria; renal venous congestion or ischemia and a reduction of filtration rate have all been implicated.[24,30]

This hypothesis became suspect when it was shown that the upright renal hemodynamic response was no different in patients with fixed orthostatic proteinuria than it was in normal subjects.[21,31] A quantitatively similar reduction of renal plasma flow and filtration rate and an elevation of filtration fraction were observed in both groups. Of these three possible hemodynamic determinants of transglomerular protein transfer, the results of clearance studies[21] suggested that the reduction of renal plasma flow that normally occurs in the upright posture was of greatest importance. For example, experimentally induced renal vasodilatation that quantitatively obliterated the usual upright reduction of renal plasma flow was accompanied by a strikingly smaller rise of protein excretion than usual. It was suggested that some function of the upright reduction of renal blood or plasma flow might secondarily permit an increased protein transfer across an altered capillary wall. According to this view, the combination of an altered capillary wall and the normal reduction of renal blood flow in the upright posture might be sufficient to effect an increased transglomerular passage of protein that readily exceeded the normal tubular reabsorptive capacity. It is possible that the secondary hemodynamic contribution to fixed orthostatic proteinuria might be similar to that occurring during the administration of angiotensin in experimental animals.[32,33]

This hypothesis is tentative, and other possibilities exist. As but one example, at least a partial contribution of an upright alteration of the renal tubular reabsorption of protein has not yet been excluded. Alternatively, increased capillary permeability to plasma proteins during standing might be mediated via a direct effect of certain humoral agents on an altered capillary wall, agents whose release is also increased by postural changes. Such a role has been suggested for renin, angiotensin, and circulating vasoactive amines because of their capacity to produce proteinuria in animals.[32–36]

Whatever the role of altered glomerular structure is in the pathogenesis of fixed orthostatic proteinuria, only long-term prospective studies can determine its clinical significance. A 20-year follow-up study of young men with an initial diagnosis of fixed orthostatic proteinuria has just been completed. Eighty-one percent still exhibited some pattern of proteinuria at 5 years, 49% at 10 years, but only 17% at 20 years.[37] Evidence of renal functional impairment or progressive renal disease had not appeared in any patient. The prevalence of other diseases known to be associated with kidney disease, such as hypertension and diabetes mellitus, was observed with a frequency no greater than that in the general population. Furthermore, there was no relationship between the initial renal histology and the subsequent pattern of renal function or proteinuria. In short, the 20-year prognosis of young men with fixed and reproducible orthostatic proteinuria is excellent. A similarly benign course has also been described by other observers over the intermediate term of 5 to 10 years.[27,38,39]

The significance of the subtle glomerular alterations that were found initially in 45% of such patients is uncertain, but the decreasing prevalence of proteinuria and the preservation of normal renal function at 20 years suggest that the glomerular findings were not a manifestation of progressive renal disease. It is also known that none of the patients has yet received financial assistance from the federal government for the treatment of end-stage renal disease. Until more time elapses, however, one cannot exclude the possibility that renal function may yet deteriorate in those few patients who still had proteinuria at 20 years. It is of interest that proteinuria was noted at 20 years in a few patients who were protein-negative at 10 years of follow-up.[37] This suggested that a negative qualitative test for protein at any given time may reflect the impact of many factors that are known to influence urine protein excretion and its qualitative detection other than any permanent resolution of the proteinuric process. Further follow-up should perhaps continue, even for those who currently appear to be protein-negative.

Taken together, these findings suggest that fixed and reproducible orthostatic proteinuria does not necessarily represent a transient condition of adolescence; albeit now less likely, in a few patients it may still reflect the earliest expression of future renal disease. Continued observation is necessary to establish the course in any individual patient, but at least the 20-year outlook is excellent.

Virtually no long-term follow-up data are available in patients with transient orthostatic proteinuria, but most believe that the prognosis of patients with this finding is excellent.[14] In many such patients, transient episodes of orthostatic proteinuria may reflect nothing more than fever, exercise, or exposure to environmental factors such as heat or cold. Indeed, it is likely that this form of upright proteinuria may derive simply from a transient and exaggerated renal hemodynamic response to these or other stimuli.

Renal biopsy specimens have now been examined from patients in each of five descriptive categories of isolated proteinuria: persistent or intermittent proteinuria (defined on sequential routine urinalysis without control of body posture)[1,4,5]; constant proteinuria during both recumbent and upright postures[7]; and transient[11] or fixed orthostatic proteinuria as defined during appropriate postural maneuvers.[7,9] In four of the five categories examined so far, a widely varying incidence of "definite" histological alterations has been reported (about 10% to 70%), all of which have been sufficiently distinct to warrant a firm histological diagnosis of kidney disease ("definite" histological alterations have not yet been reported in patients with transient orthostatic proteinuria). The lesions themselves have been extremely heterogeneous, and a consistent relationship with a given pattern of proteinuria has not been observed. The incidence of definite renal pathology has been highest (about 40% to 70%) in patients with patterns of persistent, intermittent, or constant proteinuria,[1,4,7,40] whereas a much lower figure (about 10%) has been found in patients with fixed orthostatic proteinuria (Table I).[9] In other patients from each of these groups, the incidence of disparate but minimal alterations has been similarly variable (about 10% to 70%). In still others, perhaps most frequently in patients with transient or fixed orthostatic proteinuria, the renal architecture has appeared entirely normal on light microscopy,[10,11] although subtle architectural "defects" of the glomerulus have been described on electron microscopy in a few patients.[10,28]

It seems safe to conclude that with the possible exception of transient orthostatic proteinuria, (1) each of these qualitative patterns of proteinuria may be associated with a broad spectrum of histological findings ranging from normal renal architecture to definite evidence of disease; (2) a similarly heterogeneous display of underlying renal pathology or architectural alteration occurs in each type, but the frequency of definite disease is lowest by far in patients with transient or fixed orthostatic proteinuria; and (3) no absolute relationship exists between the type of proteinuria and the presence or absence of renal pathology. Renal biopsy remains the only means of distinguishing between the patient with structural evidence of kidney disease and the one without.

Unfortunately, the description of definite pathological alterations *per se* does not provide any necessary insight into their actual clinical significance as a cause of subsequent morbidity or mortality. One still must determine whether a particular lesion is static, resolving, or progressing. In view of the marked diversity of the underlying renal pathology, it is illogical to expect that all patients will follow an identical clinical course. Prospective studies are required.

An initial examination and infrequent follow-up (every 1 to 2 years) is encouraged in patients whose isolated proteinuria is found to be persistent. A complete evaluation of patients with intermittent or transient patterns can often be deferred. Evaluation of patients with persistent patterns should include a thorough physical examination, quantification of the daily protein excretion, renal ultrasonography, and measurement of the endogenous creatinine clearance. Renal biopsy should not be undertaken unless there is a distinct change in the clinical course such as an abrupt and definite increase in daily protein excretion, the appearance of distinct and persistent abnormalities of the urine sediment, or a deterioration of renal function.

It is interesting to speculate that a persistent pattern of qualitative proteinuria over several years—whether it be persistent, intermittent, fixed or transient orthostatic, or constant in type—might be attended by an important incidence of underlying renal pathology,[5-10,14] In fact, it would not be surprising to observe different qualitative types or patterns of proteinuria in the same patient at different times over a relatively long period, because the detection and magnitude of proteinuria depend on the simultaneous interaction of many variables (for example, body posture, urine concentration, and the natural history of an underlying disease process).[41] Depending on the relationship between the lower limits of qualitative urine protein detection and the changing influences on urine protein excretion, an everchanging pattern of qualitative proteinuria may emerge. At various times, a patient may exhibit intermittent or transient orthostatic proteinuria, or perhaps it may be fixed for a variable period.[41] Eventually, quantitative protein excretion may rise sufficiently to permit its qualitative detection in both recumbent and upright specimens; that is, the proteinuria becomes constant.

Some patients may move through this sequence so explosively that constant proteinuria seems to exist from the very onset of disease. In others, the disease may progress so slowly that a variable but generally orthostatic pattern is observed for years. Eventually, if the underlying disease progresses sufficiently, protein excretion may rise during recumbency and yield a pattern of constant proteinuria; alternatively, the disease process may heal, and proteinuria will disappear completely. Considerations such as these should underscore the difficulties that beset any attempt to relate a given clinical observation to any particular qualitative pattern of proteinuria. Nevertheless, although the long-term prognosis still must be regarded with reservations in a few patients, their 20-year outlook is excellent as long as a persistent qualitative pattern of proteinuria is the sole or isolated alteration.

REFERENCES

1. Antoine B, Symvoulidis A, Dardenne M: La stabilite evolutive des etats de proteinurie permanente isolee. *Nephron* 6:526–536, 1969
2. Antoine B, Symvoulidis A, Dardenne M, et al: L'etat de proteinurie permanente isolee: I. Diversite histologique. *Presse Med* 77:9–14, 1969
3. Manuel Y, Revillard JP, Francois R, et al: Trace proteinuria, in Manuel Y, Revillard JP, Betuel H (eds): *Proteins in Normal and Pathological Urine*. Basel, S Karger, 1970, pp 198–208
4. Morel-Maroger L, Leroux-Robert C, Richet G: Renal histology in 30 cases of isolated proteinuria: Frequency of hyaline and fibrinoid deposits in renal arterioles. *Israel J Med Sci* 3:98–105, 1967
5. Muth RG: Asymptomatic mild intermittent proteinuria: A percutaneous renal biopsy study. *Arch Intern Med* 115:569–574, 1965
6. Pollak VW, Pirani CL, Muehrcke RC, et al: Asymptomatic persistent proteinuria: Studies by renal biopsies. *Guy's Hosp Rep* 107:353–372, 1958
7. Phillippi PJ, Reynolds J, Yamauchi H, et al: Persistent proteinuria in asymptomatic individuals: Renal biopsy studies on 50 patients. *Mil Med* 131:1311–1317, 1966
8. Revillard JP, Fries D, Salle B, et al: Proteinuria in glomerular disease, in Manuel Y, Revillard JP, Betuel H (eds): *Proteins in Normal and Pathological Urine*. Basel, S Karger, 1970, pp 188–197
9. Robinson RR, Glover SN, Phillippi PJ, et al: Fixed and reproducible orthostatic proteinuria: I. Light microscopic studies of the kidney. *Am J Pathol* 39:291–306, 1961
10. Robinson RR, Ashworth CT, Glover SN, et al: Fixed and reproducible and orthostatic proteinuria: II. Electron and microscopic study of renal biopsy specimens from five cases. *Am J Pathol* 39:405–417, 1961
11. Sinniah R, Law CH, Pivee HS: Glomerular lesions in patients with asymptomatic persistent and orthostatic proteinuria discovered on routine medical examination. *Clin Nephrol* 7:1–14, 1977

12. King SE: Albuminuria in renal diseases: II. Preliminary observations on the clinical course of patients with orthostatic proteinuria. NY State J Med 59:825-835, 1959
13. King SE: Diastolic hypertension and chronic proteinuria. Am J Cardiol 9:669-674, 1962
14. Levitt JI: The prognostic significance of proteinuria in young college students. Ann Intern Med 66:685-696, 1967
15. Diehl HS, McKinlay CA: Albuminuria in college men. Arch Intern Med 49:45-55, 1932
16. Wolman IJ: The incidence, causes and intermittency of proteinuria in young men. Am J Med Sci 210:86-100, 1945
17. Lyall A: The classification of cases of albuminuria. Br Med J 2:113-117, 1941
18. Burden HJ: Persistent functional albuminuria. Am J Med Sci 188:242-247, 1934
19. Derow HA: The diagnostic value of serial measurements of albuminuria in ambulatory patients. N Engl J Med 227:827-830, 1942
20. King SE: Patterns of protein excretion by the kidney. Ann Intern Med 42:296-308, 1955
21. Robinson RR, Lecocq FR, Phillippi PJ, et al: Fixed and reproducible orthostatic proteinuria: III. Effect of induced renal hemodynamic alterations upon urinary protein excretion. J Clin Invest 42:100-110, 1963
22. Robinson RR, Glenn WG: Fixed and reproducible orthostatic proteinuria: IV. Urinary albumin excretion in healthy human subjects in the recumbent and upright positions. J Lab Clin Med 64:717-721, 1964
23. Mery JP, Berger J, Milhaud A, et al: La proteinurie orthostatique: A propos de 300 observations. Rev Prat (Paris) 11:3115-3118, 1961
24. Bull GM: Postural proteinuria. Clin Sci 7:77-108, 1948
25. Fishberg AM: Orthostatic proteinuria, in Hypertension and Nephritis, ed 5. Philadelphia, Lea & Febiger, 1954, pp 396-407
26. Prince CL: Orthostatic albuminuria. J Urol 50:608-615, 1954
27. Thompson AL, Durrett RR, Robinson RR: Fixed and reproducible orthostatic proteinuria: VI. Results of a 10-year follow-up evaluation. Ann Intern Med 73:235-244, 1970
28. Ruckley VA, MacDonald MK, MacLean PR, et al: Glomerular ultrastructure and function in postural proteinuria. Nephron 3:153-166, 1966
29. Lang K, Treser G, Sagel I, et al: Routine immunohistology in renal diseases. Ann Intern Med 64:25-36, 1966
30. Greiner T, Henry JP: Mechanism of postural proteinuria. JAMA 157:1373-1378, 1955
31. King SE, Baldwin DS: Renal hemodynamics during erect lordosis in normal man and subjects with orthostatic proteinuria. Proc Soc Exp Biol Med 86:634-638, 1954
32. Eisenbach GM, Van Liew JB, Boylan JW: Effect of angiotensin on the filtration of protein in the rat kidney: A micropuncture study. Kidney Int 8:80-87, 1975
33. Bohrer MP, Deen WM, Robertson CR, et al: Mechanism of angiotensin II-induced proteinuria in the rat. Am J Physiol 2:F13-F21, 1977
34. Lathem W: Renal circulatory dynamics and urinary protein excretion during infusions of l-norepinephrine and l-epinephrine in patients with renal disease. J Clin Invest 36:1277-1285, 1957
25. Tobian L, Nason P: The augmentation of proteinuria by an acute sodium depletion that stimulates the secretion of renin. J Clin Invest 43:1301-1309, 1964
36. Montoliu J, Botey A, Torras A, et al: Renin-induced massive proteinuria in man. Clin Nephrol 11:267-271, 1979
37. Springberg PD, Garrett LE, Thompson AL, et al: Fixed and reproducible orthostatic proteinuria: Results of a 20-year follow-up study. Ann Intern Med 97:516-519, 1982
38. Chaptal J, Jean R, Bonnet H, et al: Etude histologique du rein dans 33 cas de proteinurie isolee de l'enfant. Arch Fr Pediatr 23:385-390, 1966

39. Lagrue G, Bariety J, Druet PH, et al: Les divers types de proteinuries, in *Les Proteinuries*. Paris, Sandoz, 1969, pp 1–17
40. McLaine PN, Drummond KN: Benign persistent asymptomatic proteinuria. *Pediatrics* 46:548–552, 1970
41. Robinson RR: Isolated proteinuria in asymptomatic patients. *Kidney Int* 18:395–406, 1980

Part II

Clinical Expressions of Proteinuria

Clinicians seek to associate clinical signs with structural abnormalities as a basis for the logical practice of medicine. Nephrologists have struggled with this process in their attempt to relate specific proteinuric syndromes to glomerular or tubular pathological findings. Complicating this interpretive process has been the disjointed and sometimes conflicting findings from light, fluorescence, and electron microscopy. Over the past decade, however, valid connections between anatomic lesions and response to therapy have been established. Specific therapy, it has been learned, may alter the natural history of the underlying histological lesion. As examples of incompletely understood though nevertheless effective therapeutic regimens, one could cite the use of glucocorticoids or cytotoxic drugs (cyclophosphamide, chlorambucil, azathioprine), singly or in combination, to halt (and sometimes reverse) nephron destruction, resulting in lessening of proteinuria in several forms of glomerulonephritis.

The first four chapters of this part review the relationship between specific pathological lesions and proteinuria in diverse entities, including lipoid nephrosis (minimal-change nephrotic syndrome), renal allografts in diabetics, renal allografts in nondiabetics, and "nonmedical" proteinuria. Each chapter details pathogenetic mechanisms, immunopathology, and treatment of the specific entity.

Hayslett, who more than a decade ago observed the progression of lipoid nephrosis to renal insufficiencies, reviews diagnostic criteria and therapy of minimal-change disease as distinguished from glomerular focal glomerulosclerosis. A rich data resource is provided in patient follow-ups for 16 years, including interpretation of prospective controlled trials with cyclophosphamide and chlorambucil. It is evident that a satisfactory solution to management of minimal-change/focal glomerular sclerosis in nephrosis is not yet available. Baldwin, in a more encouraging note, recounts the reversibility of renal failure in minimal-change nephrotic syndrome. He describes the course of 15 patients, nine older than 60 years, with renal failure of 10 days' to 2 weeks' duration in whom renal biopsy authenticated a minimal-change glomerular lesion. According to Baldwin, induction of diuresis, whether by diuretics or remission, is crucial to recovery. It is hypothesized that a washout of proteinaceous fluid from glomeruli and tubules will reduce interstitial pressure and restore normal vasoactive responses, thereby reestablishing urine flow.

The next two reports examine the special case of proteinuria in transplanted kidneys. Friedman and associates, in an elegant study, surveyed the prevalence and significance of proteinuria in 47 renal allograft recipients up to 82 months post-transplantation. Of these, 15 recipients were diabetic pretransplant. Proteinuria was nearly universal in all recipients. Urinary protein excretion ranged between 0.14 and 1.0 g/day with no reported difference between diabetic and nondiabetic patients. Interestingly, the rate of bacteriuria in all recipients was very low (6.4%), suggesting that urinary infection is of minor import in the genesis of proteinuria in this setting. In a matching report, Stenzel and associates communicate their experience with proteinuria in 1000 kidney transplants over 20 years at the New York Hospital. The authors' analysis indicates that proteinuria after a kidney transplant may be multifactorial. The presence of proteinuria >3 g/day predicts loss of the renal allograft within 5 years. Renal donors, it is noted in the initial report of an ongoing study, may become hypertensive and proteinuric; the significance of these findings is unknown. Godec addressed nonmedical urological causes of proteinuria. He reports on the association between malignancies and benign tumors and proteinuria. Proteinuria should be regarded as an "early messenger for a multitude of urological disorders," he suggests. About 11% of new-onset adult nephrotics have an underlying cancer—a chilling abnegation of the concept of "benign nephrosis."

M.M.A.

6

Clinical Spectrum of Lipoid Nephrosis

JOHN P. HAYSLETT

INTRODUCTION

The term lipoid nephrosis is used to denote the nephrotic syndrome produced by a glomerulopathy characterized by normal or minimal histopathological changes by light microscopy. By electron and immunofluorescent microscopy there is generalized effacement of foot processes of epithelial cells and negligible deposits of immunoglobulins and complement. Since neither the etiology or the pathogenesis of lipoid nephrosis is established, lipoid nephrosis can be considered as a syndrome with some variants in regard to pathology and clinical characteristics. Some years ago we suggested that focal glomerulosclerosis was one such variant, and in this review we consider lipoid nephrosis under the two general headings of minimal-change disease and focal glomerulosclerosis.

MINIMAL-CHANGE DISEASE

The diagnosis of minimal-change disease is established by the pattern of histopathological changes found on renal biopsy. The WHO classification includes the features shown in Table I.[1] This is the most common cause of nephrotic syndrome in children and has a male predominance. In preschool children, minimal-change nephrotic syndrome accounted for more than 90% of cases of nephrotic syndrome in 66 unselected patients reported by Churg, Habib, and White; after the age of 6–7 years, the incidence fell gradually until adolescence, when it accounted for approximately one-half of cases.[2] In adult patients this

JOHN P. HAYSLETT • Department of Medicine, Section of Nephrology, Yale University School of Medicine, New Haven, Connecticut 06510.

Table I. WHO Classification of Lipoid Nephrosis

Glomerular classification	Light microscopy	Electron microscopy	Immunofluorescence microscopy
Minimal change	Minor changes of epithelial cells, sometimes with: 1. Increase in mesangial cells (3 cells/area) 2. Widening of mesangium (up to twice normal) 3. Occasional splitting, wrinkling, or thickening 4. Generalized increase in thickness of capillary basement membrane (up to twice normal for age)	Loss or effacement of epithelial foot processes	0 or ±IgM, IgG
Focal and segmental hyalinosis and sclerosis	Focal segmental hyalinosis and sclerosis, sometimes with: 1. Mild to moderate widening and cellularity 2. Tubular atrophy 3. Interstitial fibrosis and inflammation	Loss or effacement of epithelial foot processes	IgM and C3 localized to sclerotic areas and sometimes the mesangium

pathological entity is found in about 20% of cases of nephrotic syndrome caused by a primary glomerulopathy, and this frequency persists beyond the age of 60.[3] Most children with minimal-change disease have a relapsing course. In the series of 61 patients described by Siegel and associates,[4] 84% had at least one recurrence, and in the White series the incidence was 92%.[5] As shown in Fig. 1, although only 23% of relapsing patients remained free of recurrence during the first year, approximately one-half of the group was in remission during each of the subsequent 6 years. Although the proportion of patients who continued to experience relapse decreased further with time, 20% continued to have relapses as long as 15 years after onset, with preservation of renal function. It is generally assumed that in children the syndrome spontaneously disappears by adulthood, since nephrotic syndrome is uncommon in adults with a history of the childhood disorder. There is less information on the likelihood of recurrence in adults, but the incidence appears to be less than in children, at about 30%.[6]

There is less data on the natural course of minimal-change disease in children prior to the era of antibiotic and glucocorticoid therapy. In a follow-up of 62 children who were treated before 1950, reported by Arneil and Lam, the survival rate was approximately 50%, and death resulted primarily from sepsis.[7] In recent reports on the clinical course modified by glucocorticoid therapy, approximately 2% to 4% died of causes related to renal disease, either from renal failure or shock resulting from vascular collapse.[4,8] It is of interest that in adult patients Black and associates reported a spontaneous remission rate of approximately 75% by 2 to 3 years after onset.[9] Although controversy invariably envelops any attempt to distinguish minimal-change nephrotic syndrome from focal glomerulosclerosis, it seems probable that some patients with typical minimal-change disease eventually progress to chronic glomerulosclerosis and renal failure. This type of course was initially described by Hayslett and associates in three cases with minimal-change disease by biopsy who exhibited a polyrelapsing, steroid-sensitive course for 2 to 16 years before sclerosing changes were evident by biopsy.[10] It was assumed that the initial disease was minimal change because of the persistent steroid responsiveness in addition to the biopsy findings.

Despite the absence of severe renal histopathological findings, renal insufficiency may occur during relapse in some patients with lipoid nephrosis. In children, a blood urea nitrogen value >20 mg/dl was reported in 27% of 52 children in the absence of concurrent steroid therapy.[4] In adult patients, especially in the elderly, severe renal insufficiency has been described during relapse, and, since recovery of renal function occurred during diuretic treatment, the decline in glomerular filtration rate was ascribed to intrarenal edema.[11]

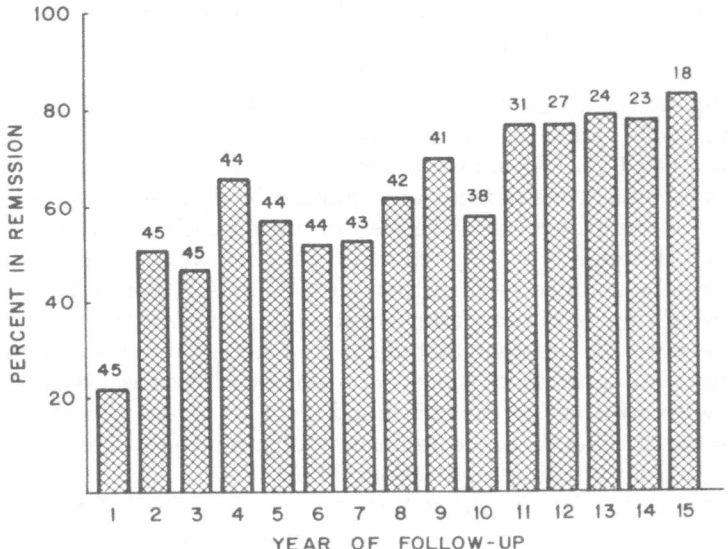

Figure 1. Percentage of relapsing patients who were free of relapse during each individual year of follow-up. Number of patients remaining in the group during each follow-up year is indicated at the top of each bar.

Minimal-change nephrotic syndrome is characterized by a complete clinical remission following glucocorticoid or alkylating drug therapy. In the series reported by White and associates, for example, 93 of 95 children (98%) responded to steroid treatment during the initial episode,[5] and most patients continue to exhibit the same pattern of response even after many years of a polyrelapsing course. Treatment usually includes prednisone in a dose of 2 mg/kg for approximately 4 to 6 weeks, and response occurs on average within 10 ± 1 days. In the report of the International Study of Kidney Disease in Children (ISKDC), a small number (3.8%) of children with normal glomerular histology who were nonresponders by 8 weeks eventually became free of proteinuria by 1 year.[8] Therapy with cytotoxic agents has been employed primarily in children with frequently relapsing minimal-change nephrotic syndrome rather than as initial treatment. In prospective controlled trials, both cyclophosphamide and chlorambucil have been demonstrated to induce long-lasting remissions compared to continued use of prednisone alone.[12,13] Concern for the possible adverse effects of these agents on reproductive and endocrine functions of the gonad, however, has limited their use to the small group of cases with very frequent relapses, to patients with unacceptable side effects from glucocorticoids, and to steroid resistant patients.[14] Alkylating drugs have been administered as initial therapy in older adults, however, with good results.

Although an abnormality in T-cell function has been proposed as the cause of minimal-change nephrotic syndrome,[15] the pathogenesis of this disorder remains unknown. It is of interest, therefore, that the typical glomerular findings have been found in patients with Hodgkin's disease[16] and during the administration of nonsteroidal antiinflammatory drugs.[17] In Hodgkin's disease, the normal reactive lymphocytes associated with the Reed–Sternberg cells are predominantly T cells, and an interstitial infiltration composed of T cells was reported in drug-induced cases of minimal-change nephrotic syndrome.

FOCAL GLOMERULOSCLEROSIS

Rich initially described focal deposits of hyaline in glomerular tufts, limited to juxtamedullary glomeruli, in seven children who died in the early phase of nephrotic syndrome.[18] Subsequently, Churg and associates described focal glomerulosclerosis in 9% of 127 children evaluated in the ISKDC project.[2] This lesion was described as glomerular sclerosis in a focal and segmental distribution, which in the advanced stage showed partly or completely sclerosed glomeruli with accompanying tubular atrophy and interstitial inflammatory changes. By electron microscopy, extensive effacement of foot processes was found, as in the minimal-change lesion. Subsequent analyses in children[5] and adults[19] have reported that the lesion of focal glomerulosclerosis, when diagnosed near the onset of disease, was associated with nonresponsiveness to steroids and cytotoxic drugs in the great majority of cases and a high frequency of progressive renal failure. Predicted survival rates were estimated to range from 18% to 50%.[20,21] On the basis of what appeared to be distinctive clinical-pathological features, some authors proposed that focal glomerulosclerosis was a separate nosological disease entity.[22]

Our laboratory, however, presented a select group of patients that suggested that focal glomerulosclerosis may be part of the spectrum of lipoid nephrosis, which has a wide range of histological and clinical features, as shown in Table II.[23] In this report of six children with normal glomeruli by light and electron microscopy, four were resistant to steroids. Although sclerotic lesions in deep portions of cortex may have been missed by biopsy, all six exhibited a complete remission while on cyclophosphamide treatment. A second group of six patients were steroid dependent, and normal glomeruli were found by light micros-

Table II. Minimal Change and Focal Sclerotic Lesions in Lipoid Nephrosis

Histopathology	Number	Response to steroids	Response to cytoxan	Duration of disease
Minimal change (light, EM)	6	2/6	6/6	2.7 years
Minimal change (light), focal sclerosis (EM)	6	6/6	6/6	10.2 years
Focal glomerulosclerosis (light, EM)	10	7/10	5/6	13.8 years

copy, but early evidence of glomerular sclerosis was evident on ultra-structural examination. Finally, ten patients with onset of nephrotic syndrome at less than 6 years of age and a steroid-sensitive, polyrelapsing course for 3 to 17 years had focal sclerotic lesions in glomeruli and tubular atrophy; seven of these ten patients were responsive to steroid and/or cytotoxic agents at the time of biopsy. These observations demonstrated a broad spectrum of clinicopathological relationships in the nephrotic syndrome of childhood and provided further evidence that in some patients focal glomerulosclerosis may evolve from a minimal-change lesion. Subsequent experience has served to corroborate this conclusion.

Table III shows the results of 38 children with a steroid-dependent polyrelapsing course who were biopsied a mean of 6 years after onset.[24] Eleven of 38, or 29%, had focal glomerulosclerosis, and, in addition to steroid sensitivity, all 11 experienced a complete clinical remission on cyclophosphamide therapy. Additional evidence for the wide spectrum of histological changes in lipoid nephrosis is shown in Table IV, taken from a report by the ISKDC.[8] The distribution of lesions on initial biopsy, obtained near onset of disease, included focal glomerular obsolescence (FGO) in 25% of 389 children and focal tubular changes (FTC) in 8%. By the criteria employed in this analysis, these lesions were included under the heading of minimal-change nephrotic syndrome. Within 8 weeks of steroid therapy, a complete clinical remission occurred in 92% with focal glomerular obsolescence and 86% with focal tubular changes. In patients with a Nil lesion, in contrast, the response rate was 95%. After 52 weeks of follow-up, however, there was no difference in the remission rate between the groups with histopathological changes and patients with a Nil lesion. Since this report regarded diffuse mesangial hypercellularity as a variant of minimal-change nephrotic syndrome, it is of interest that whereas only 55% of cases were initial responders, nearly 90% were protein-free by 1 year, presumably from spontaneous remission. These results concerning diffuse mesangial hypercellularity, which indi-

Table III. Steroid-Dependent Polyrelapsing Course in Children[a]

	Minimal change	Meangial proliferative	Focal glomerulosclerosis
Renal Bx, number	18	9	11
Response to cytoxan	100%	100%	100%
Relapse (4–6 yr)	22%	56%	73%

[a]Correlation of renal histopathology and response to treatment in 38 children for a mean of 6 years. From Siegel et al.,[24] with permission.

cate a high rate of steroid responsiveness and a tendency toward spontaneous improvement, agree with other reports in which this lesion was not regarded as a variant of minimal-change nephrotic syndrome.[25]

The ominous outlook for focal sclerosis has also changed, compared to initial reports, as experience has accumulated. Mongeau and associates, for example, have described the clinical course of 25 children with focal glomerulosclerosis and seven with focal global glomerulosclerosis.[26] Twenty-five percent of cases with focal glomerulosclerosis responded to steroids, as did all treated patients with focal global glomerulosclerosis. The actuarial curve for the former group of patients predicted that 32% developed renal failure within 4 years of onset. In contrast to early reports, however, which predicted a general tendency towards progressive renal failure, renal function remained stable in 68% of cases for as long as 19 years of observation.

Taking all of this experience together, it becomes apparent that (1) classification of the histological variants of lipoid nephrosis includes a wide spectrum of changes, (2) transformation of minimal-change disease to focal glomerulosclerosis occurs in some patients, and (3) a spectrum of clinical patterns correlates with focal glomerular sclerosis, tubular atrophy, and mesangial hypercellularity. It seems clear that normal histo-

Table IV. Percentages of Nonresponders to Steroids in Children with "Minimal-Change Nephrotic Syndrome," ISKDC study

Time after starting treatment (weeks)	Histological categories[a] (%)					
	Nil	FGO	MMT	FTC	MMH	DMH
8	4.7	7.8	6.3	14.3	14.8	45.5
16	1.9	4.4	6.3	10.7	14.8	27.3
52	0.9	2.2	0.0	3.6	7.4	9.1

[a]Abbreviations: Nil, normal structure; FGO, focal glomerular obsolescence; MMT, mild mesangial thickening; FTC, focal tubular changes; MMH, mild mesangial hypercellularity; DMH, diffuse mesangial hypercellularity.

logical findings or minor histopathological changes by light microscopy are associated with a high frequency of steroid responsiveness and a favorable long-term outlook, even with a polyrelapsing clinical course. The presence of focal sclerotic lesions early in the course of disease correlates with a higher incidence of resistance to therapy and significant propensity for progression to renal failure. In cases in which focal glomerular sclerosis evolves from a minimal lesion after several years of disease, however, clinical experience indicates a high degree of responsiveness to treatment and preservation of renal function.

The great French neurologist Jean Marten Charcot once observed that clinical medicine is made of anomalies whereas nosography is a description of phenomena that occur regularly. Lipoid nephrosis is no exception to this rule of exceptions. Since there is no distinctive clinical course for patients with focal glomerulosclerosis, there appears to be no advantage in regarding this lesion as representing a separate nosological disease. The data suggest, therefore, a broad spectrum of histopathological and clinical features in lipoid nephrosis, as shown in Fig. 2. Recognition of the relationships within this spectrum will continue to provide guidelines in managing patients with nephrotic syndrome until future studies delineate specific markers for individual diseases included within the syndrome of lipoid nephrosis.

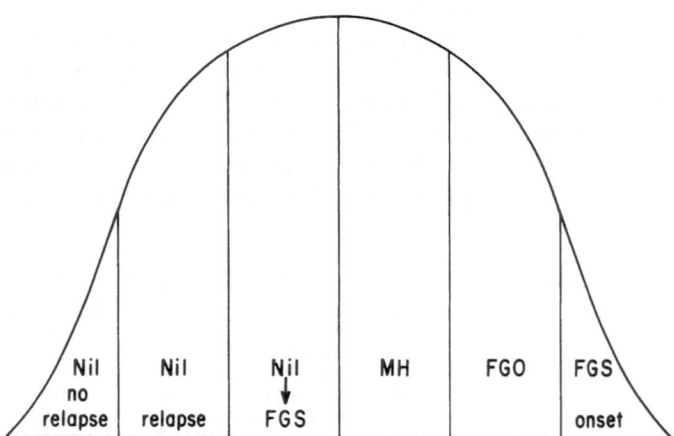

Figure 2. Proposed histopathological spectrum of lipoid nephrosis. Nil = normal glomerular histology; FGS = focal glomerulosclerosis; MH = increase in mesangial cells with or without an increase in mesangial matrix; FGO = focal glomerular obsolescence.

REFERENCES

1. Churg J, Sobin LH: *Renal Disease: Classification and Atlas of Glomerular Disease*. Tokyo, New York, Igaku-Shoin, 1982, pp 35–53
2. Churg J, Habib R, White RHR: Pathology of the nephrotic syndrome in children. *Lancet* 1:1299–1304, 1970
3. Zech P, Colon PH, Deteix P, et al: The nephrotic syndrome in adults aged over 60: Etiology, evaluation and treatment of 76 cases. *Clin Nephrol* 18:232–236, 1982
4. Siegel NJ, Goldberg B, Krassner LS, et al: Long-term follow-up of children with steroid-responsive nephrotic syndrome. *J Pediatr* 81:251–1972
5. White RHR, Glasgow EF, Mills RJ: Clinicopathological study of nephrotic syndrome in childhood. *Lancet* 1:1353–1359, 1979
6. Hopper J, Ryan P, Lee JC, et al: Lipoid nephrosis in 31 adult patients: Renal biopsy study by light, electron, and fluorescence microscopy with experience in treatment. *Medicine* 49:321–341, 1970
7. Arneil GC, Lam CN: Long-term assessment of steroid therapy in childhood nephrosis. *Lancet 2:819–821, 1966*
8. *International Study of Kidney Disease in Children: Primary nephrotic syndrome in children: Clinical significance of histopathologic variants of minimal change and of diffuse mesangial hypercellularity.* Kidney Int 20:765–771, 1981
9. Black DAK, Rose G, Brewer DB: Controlled trial of prednisone in adult patients with the nephrotic syndrome. *Br J Med* 2:431–436, 1970
10. Hayslett JP, Krassner LS, Bensch KG, et al: Progression of 'lipoid nephrosis' to renal insufficiency. *N Engl J Med* 281:181–187, 1969
11. Lowenstein J, Schacht RG, Baldwin DS: Renal failure in minimal change nephrotic syndrome. *Am J Med* 70:227–233, 1981
12. International Study of Kidney Disease in Children: Prospective, controlled trial of cyclophosphamide therapy in children with the nephrotic syndrome. *Lancet* 2:423–427, 1974
13. Grupe WE: Chlorambucil in steroid-dependent nephrotic syndrome. *J Pediatr* 82:598–606, 1973
14. Qureski MSA, Pennington JH, Goldsmith HJ, et al: Cyclophosphamide therapy and sterility. *Lancet* 2:1290–1291, 1972
15. Shalhoub RJ: Pathogenesis of lipoid nephrosis: A disorder of T-cell function. *Lancet* 2:556–560, 1974
16. Moorthy AV, Zimmerman SW, Burkholder PM: Nephrotic syndrome in Hodgkin's disease: Evidence for pathogenesis alternative to immune complex deposition. *Am J Med* 61:471–477, 1976
17. Finkelstein A, Fraley D, Stachura I, et al: Fenoprofen nephropathy: Lipoid nephrosis and interstital nephritis. *Am J Med* 72:81–87, 1982
18. Rich A: A hitherto undescribed vulnerability of the juxtamedullary glomeruli in lipoid nephrosis. *Bull Johns Hopkins Hosp* 100:173–186, 1957
19. Velosa JA, Donadio JV, Holley KE: Focal sclerosing glomerulonephropathy. A clinciopathological study. *Mayo Clin Proc* 50:121–132, 1975
20. Cameron JS, Turner DR, Ogg CS, et al: The long-term prognosis of patients with focal segmental glomerulosclerosis. *Clin Nephrol* 10:213–281, 1978
21. Habib R: Focal glomerulosclerosis. *Kidney Int* 1973:4:355–361, 1973
22. Editorial: Focal glomerulosclerosis. *Lancet* 2:367, 1972

92   John P. Hayslett

23. Siegel NJ, Kashgarian M, Spargo BH, et al: Minimal change and focal sclerotic lesions in lipoid nephrosis. *Nephron* 13:125–137, 1974
24. Siegel NJ, Gaudio KM, Krassner LS, et al: Steroid-dependent nephrotic syndrome in children: Histopathology and relapses after cyclophosphamide treatment. *Kidney Int* 19:454–459, 1981
25. Brown EA, Kirti Upadhyaya BM, Hayslett JP, et al: The clinical course of mesangial proliferative glomerulonephritis. *Medicine* 58:295–303, 1979
26. Mongeau JG, Corneille L, Robitaille P, et al: Primary nephrosis in childhood associated with focal glomerular sclerosis: Is long-term prognosis that severe? *Kidney Int* 20:743–746, 1981

7

Reversible Renal Failure in Minimal-Change Nephrotic Syndrome

DAVID S. BALDWIN

INTRODUCTION

Renal failure as it occurs in the course of chronic glomerular diseases is generally slowly progressive and irreversible and is caused by anatomic obliteration of the glomerular filtering bed by proliferation of endothelial and epithelial cells, by thickening of capillary walls, by sclerosis resulting from primary glomerular damage, or by ischemic changes related to intrarenal vascular disease. In the absence of a structural basis for glomerular obliteration in minimal-change nephrotic syndrome (MCNS), functional deterioration would not be expected to occur. However, acute renal failure in patients with the nephrotic syndrome and minimal glomerular changes has been reported by a number of observers since 1958[1-14] in a total of approximately 50 patients. Deterioration of renal function in this group of patients has generally been attributed to presumed hypovolemia secondary to hypoalbuminemia with resultant renal vasoconstriction with or without ischemic acute tubular necrosis. A minority of observers have proposed causative roles for tubular obstruction by proteinaceous casts or increased intrarenal pressure related to interstitial edema.

Aside from the fact that renal tissue has rarely shown acute tubular necrosis, features of the clinical course in the patients reported raise major questions concerning the likelihood that renal ischemia and its sequelae are responsible for functional deterioration in MCNS. Primarily, renal failure has often lasted many weeks to months, occasionally has proved to be irreversible, and in some cases has been recurrent. Further, hypovolemia has not been demonstrable in most instances, and, finally,

DAVID S. BALDWIN • Department of Medicine, New York University Medical Center, New York, New York 10016.

recovery of renal function has almost invariably coincided with induced diuresis or with remission of the nephrotic syndrome either under corticosteroid therapy or occurring spontaneously. For these reasons, it appears that an explanation other than acute tubular necrosis must be sought to account for renal failure as it occurs in the patient with nephrotic syndrome and minimal glomerular changes.

In our own experience at New York University,[11] the striking association between induction of diuresis and recovery of renal function and the finding of remarkably decreased filtration rates relative to renal plasma flow have led to the hypothesis that a reduction in net ultrafiltration pressure occurs in MCNS as a result of increased intratubular pressure, which, in turn, is responsible for reversible contraction of the filtering surface area of the glomerulus.

THE NEW YORK UNIVERSITY SERIES

Fifteen patients were hospitalized at Bellevue or at New York University Hospital with varying degrees of renal insufficiency and the nephrotic syndrome, defined as heavy proteinuria (>3.5 g/24) associated with hypoalbuminemia. Nine were over 60 years of age; the others were 15, 19, 23, 35, 46, and 54 years old. Thirteen were male.

Renal biopsy specimens were examined by light, immunofluorescence, and electron microscopic techniques as described previously.[15] Glomerular filtration rate (GFR) and renal plasma flow (RPF) were measured by standard clearance techniques using a constant infusion of inulin and p-aminohippurate. Quantitative protein excretion was determined by the biuret method.

CLINICAL FEATURES

The duration of the nephrotic syndrome prior to presentation ranged from 10 days to 12 weeks (Table I). In 13 patients, no history of prior renal disease was obtained; in patients 1 and 2, the youngest in the series, nephrotic syndrome with minimal glomerular change had been documented previously, and the present observations were made during relapses that occurred 1 and 3 years following discontinuation of corticosteroid therapy. Patients 3 and 4 were observed during two episodes, and patient 6 during three episodes of reversible renal failure. All presented with anasarca, massive proteinuria, markedly depressed serum albumin (range 0.4 to 2.4, mean 1.5 g/dl), and elevated serum

Table I. Clinical Features of Renal Failure in MCNS; Response to Therapy

Pt.	Age	Peak value before therapy						Following induced diuresis alone					Following remission of proteinuria and further diuresis				Treatment[a]
		24-h urine volume (ml)	Serum albumin (g/dl)	24-h protein excretion (g)	Wt. (lb)	BUN (mg/dl)	Creat. (mg/dl)	Serum albumin (g/dl)	24-h protein excretion (g)	Wt. (lb)	BUN (mg/dl)	Creat. (mg/dl)	24-h protein excretion (g)	Wt. (lb)	BUN (mg/dl)	Creat. (mg/dl)	
1	23	—	1.5	—	145	92	3.0	No diuresis					Trace	115	10	1.0	CS
2	15	—	0.4	—	122	76	2.6	No diuresis					Negative	106	18	0.9	CS
3b	64	700	1.7	5.7	139	73	2.3	2.3	12.0	136	32	1.4	1.3	112	15	0.8	CS,SPA
4a	66	760	1.5	9.7	156	88	2.7	2.5	7.9	139	27	1.0	2.1	112	21	0.5	CS,D,CYT,SPA
4b	66	650	1.5	5.5	133	116	3.4	2.9	3.4	121	36	1.0	1.8	119	22	0.8	CS,D,CYT,SPA
5	67	1450	2.4	11.0	185	84	2.9	3.7	14.8	167	73	1.7	2.6	165	29	1.1	CS,D,SPA
6a	81	550	1.8	5.0	194	89	4.7	1.8	4.5	158	22	1.3	0.2	161	15	1.0	CS,CYT,D
7	75	400	1.9	13.0	144	147	7.6	1.3	7.1	129	89	2.3	(2+)	129	16	1.0	CS
8	76	540	1.3	8.6	160	99	5.9	1.6	9.0	148	58	2.4	1.5		13	1.2	CS,D
6b	76	250	1.9	4.7	177	95	5.6	2.7	3.6	155	24	1.2	No remission				CS,D,SPA,CYT
6c	76	1050	1.5	5.5	171	80	6.2	1.4	7.0	149	44	1.6	No remission				CS,D,SPA,CYT
9	19	330	1.1	8.0	143	120	3.2	1.0	6.9	110	10	0.7	No remission				CYT,D
10	71	250	1.1	6.3	163	49	3.0	1.5	20	128	23	1.2	No remission				CS,D,SPA
11	54	1280	1.8	15.7	215	154	11.6	1.7	8.0	168	16	1.6	No remission				CS,D,SPA
3a	64	350	1.3	5.4	147	53	2.6	2.5	15.1	130	27	1.7	No remission				SPA
12	46	650	1.6	13.9	145	180	6.9	1.9	26.4	128	122	3.3	No remission				CS,AZA,D,SPA
13	35	900	1.0	11.5	199	105	4.5	2.2	19.7	171	33	1.9	No remission				D
14	67	150	1.6	9.4	220	138	13.4	No diuresis					No remission				CS
15	69	600	1.5	18.7	161	87	7.7	No diuresis					No remission				CS,D

[a]Treatments abbreviated as follows: CS, corticosteroid; D, diuretics; CYT, cyclophosphamide; AZA, azathioprine; SPA, salt-poor albumin.

cholesterol. Urine volume exceeded 500 ml/24 in only four of the patients who were not already receiving diuretics at the time of admission to the hospital. Urine sodium concentration was less than 10 mEq/liter in nine patients, 15 and 33 mEq/liter in two others, and was not recorded in the remaining four. The excretion fraction for sodium, measured in six patients, ranged from 0.02% to 0.17%. Microscopic hematuria was present in seven and hypertension in eight of the 15. No patient presented with hypotension or other clinical evidence of hypovolemia.

Renal insufficiency was present at the time of admission to the hospital in all 15 patients as evidenced by blood urea nitrogens (BUN) ranging from 32 to 121 mg/dl and serum creatinines from 2.3 to 9.5 mg/dl. In nine, a further increase in BUN and serum creatinine was observed during the first 1–2 weeks of hospitalization, the average serum creatinine increasing from 3.6 to 5.2 mg/dl.

PATHOLOGY

Light-microscopic examination of renal biopsy tissue, obtained within the first 2 weeks of hospitalization in all patients, revealed either no glomerular abnormalities or minimal changes characterized by increased mesangial matrix and minimal mesangial hypercellularity in 13. Immunofluorescence microscopy performed in 13 patients was negative or at most revealed the presence of faint mesangial staining for IgG. Immunoglobulins and complement were not found in peripheral capillary loops. Electron-microscopic examination, which was performed in eight, was normal except for foot process fusion; electron-dense deposits were not seen. In patient 6, a second renal biopsy was obtained during a recurrence of renal failure 27 months following the onset of MCNS and again revealed only minimal glomerular abnormalities. The remaining two patients, 7 and 11, showed glomerular abnormalities, but these proved not to account for their renal failure, which was reversible as in the other 13. In patient 7, whose serum creatinine reached a level of 7.6 mg/dl, focal segmental proliferation was seen. Global sclerosis of approximately 50% of glomeruli, the others appearing normal, was present in patient 11, whose serum creatinine decreased from 11.6 to 1.6 mg/dl during diuresis. The reversal of renal failure that followed induced diuresis in patients 7 and 11 appeared to follow the same pattern as was seen in the 13 patients in whom the diagnosis of MCNS was made; the 15 patients have therefore been considered as a group in the present report. Tubular necrosis was not seen in renal biopsy samples. In many biopsy specimens, interstitial edema, as evidenced by separation of tubules, was noted; no effort was made to estimate the degree of interstitial edema quantitatively.

Postmortem examination was performed in three patients, patients 14 and 15, who died with persistent nephrotic syndrome and renal failure after 2 months of treatment, and patient 10, who died of sepsis. Serum creatinine prior to death was 2.8 mg/dl in patient 10, 7.8 mg/dl in 13, and 10.3 mg/dl in 14 (on maintenance hemodialysis). The renal lesion was classified as "minimal change" in each and did not differ from the earlier renal biopsies. In no instance on postmortem examination of the kidney was there evidence of tubular necrosis; thrombosis of the renal veins, outside or within the kidney, was not present.

CLINICAL COURSE

An increase in filtration rate, as evidenced by a fall in BUN and serum creatinine, occurred with induction of diuresis in 13 of the 15 patients on a total of 17 occasions. Improvement in renal function accompanied diuresis whether or not remission of proteinuria and of the nephrotic syndrome subsequently occurred (Table I, Fig. 1).

The course of eight patients in whom reversal of renal failure during induction of diuresis was followed by remission of the nephrotic syndrome is shown in the upper portion of Table I and in the right panel of Fig. 1. All eight patients received corticosteroid in doses greater than 50 mg/day. Four were treated with diuretics, usually large doses of furosemide. Three patients were given, in addition, daily infusions of 25-50 of salt-poor albumin (Table I). On nine occasions (twice in patient 4), a decline in serum creatinine occurred in response to diuresis before steroid-induced remission of massive proteinuria was achieved. Weight loss averaged 15 lb. Serum creatinine fell from a mean of 4.0 mg/dl to 1.6 mg/dl during induced diuresis. Serum albumin increased following induced diuresis in some patients, but the changes were small when they did occur; serum albumin averaged 1.56 ± 0.18 g/dl prior to diuresis and 2.0 ± 0.34 g/dl following diuresis. With subsequent remission of the nephrotic syndrome, further diuresis with additional mean weight loss of 7 lb. was observed, and the decline in serum creatinine proceeded to a mean value of 0.9 mg/dl. In patient 1, no diuresis occurred prior to steroid-induced remission of the nephrotic syndrome; in him, remission of the nephrotic syndrome, diuresis, and recovery of renal function took place concomitantly.

Improvement in filtration rate occurred in response to diuresis on eight occasions in seven patients in whom ultimate remission of the

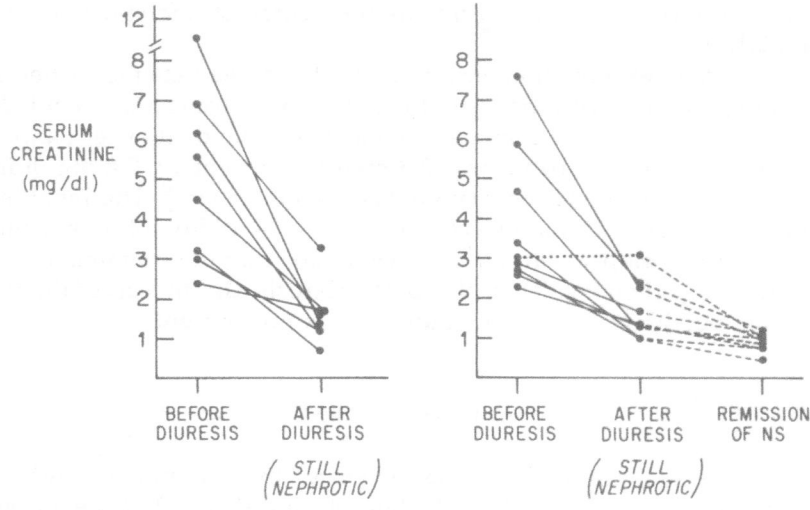

Figure 1. Reversal of renal failure during diuresis in minimal-change nephrotic syndrome (MCNS). The panel on the left depicts the responses during diuresis of seven patients with steroid-resistant nephrotic syndrome. The panel on the right depicts the responses of eight patients in whom remission of the nephrotic syndrome was induced by corticosteroid. One patient, indicated by the dashed line, was treated with corticosteroid alone and did not undergo a diuresis prior to remission of the nephrotic syndrome.

nephrotic syndrome failed to occur (Table I, lower portion, and Fig. 1, left panel). Patients 3a and 13 received no corticosteroids. In patient 3a, treatment consisted solely of dietary sodium restriction and daily infusion of 25–50 g of salt-poor albumin; serum albumin increased from 1.3 to 2.5 g/dl, and a diuresis of 17 lb ensued. Serum creatinine decreased from 2.6 to 1.7 mg/dl in association with diuresis, although protein excretion increased from 5.4 to 15.1 daily during albumin administration. Following discontinuation of albumin infusions, edema reaccumulated, and serum creatinine again increased from 1.7 to 2.3 mg/dl. Patient 13 was treated with diuretics only; diuresis of 28 lb was associated with a fall in serum creatinine from 4.5 to 1.9 mg/dl. In the remaining five patients, corticosteroid therapy was given but did not induce remission of the nephrotic syndrome; diuresis was achieved by administration of large doses of furosemide and spironolactone together with daily infusion of salt-poor albumin in four. Diuresis with an average weight loss of 26 lb (range 17–36) occurred over a period of several weeks and was associated temporally with an improvement in filtration rate, serum creatinine falling from a mean of 3.7 (range 2.6 to 11.6 mg/dl) to 1.6 mg/dl despite persistence of massive proteinuria. Changes in serum albumin concentration were small, averaging 1.41 ± 0.12 g/dl before and 1.86 ± 0.20 g/dl following diuresis; in no patient did serum albumin exceed 2.7 g/dl.

Patients 14 and 15 failed to undergo either diuresis or remission of the nephrotic syndrome. Both died with persistent renal failure, complicated terminally by infection and gastrointestinal hemorrhage.

RENAL HEMODYNAMICS

Glomerular filtration rate (GFR) and effective renal plasma flow (RPF) were measured using standard clearance techniques in six patients. The GFR was markedly reduced, ranging from 6.6 to 29.4 ml/min (Table II). The clearance of PAH was moderately reduced, ranging from 199 to 410 ml/min. Filtration fractions (C_{IN}/C_{PAH}) were remarkably low, ranging from 0.03 to 0.095. In patient 3a, following initial measurement of GFR and RPF, daily infusion of salt-poor albumin (25–50 g/day) was given for 14 days. Serum albumin increased from an initial value of 1.3 g/dl to 2.5 g/dl, and diuresis occurred despite even heavier proteinuria. Repeat hemodynamic measurements revealed an increase in GFR from 29.4 to 41.5 ml/min, in RPF from 310 to 397 ml/min, and in filtration fraction from 0.095 to 0.105.

DISCUSSION

The New York University Medical Center observations document the occurrence of renal insufficiency on 19 occasions in 15 patients with the nephrotic syndrome and minimal glomerular changes. Renal failure was not severe in most of our patients, serum creatinine ranging from 2.3 to 7.6 mg/dl in 16 episodes and exceeding this value on only three occasions. Although most of the patients tended to be oliguric, reduction in urine output was interpreted mostly to reflect avid sodium and water retention as a manifestation of severe nephrotic syndrome rather than oliguria related to glomerular insufficiency. In support of this interpretation was the response to diuretics on all but two occasions, which in turn was followed by improvement in renal function. The failure of two patients to respond to diuretics and their requirement for maintenance hemodialysis are similar to the courses of approximately 35 other patients who have been reported in the literature with MCNS and oliguric renal failure. The patients described could not be diuresed and recovered renal function only after many weeks or months on hemodialysis, when

Table II. Glomerular Filtration Rate and Renal Plasma Flow in MCNS

Patient	Serum creatinine (mg/dl)	C~INULIN~ (ml/min)	C~PAH~ (ml/min)	Filtration fraction
6	5.1	6.6	199	0.03
4	2.0	13.0	265	0.06
10	2.8	15.0	208	0.07
13	4.2	23.0	410	0.06
8	2.4	22.0	258	0.08
3	2.4	29.4	310	0.095
3[a]	1.7	41.5	397	0.105

[a]Following induced diuresis.

remission of the nephrotic syndrome finally was induced or occurred spontaneously.

It appears from our own experience that with moderate renal failure in MCNS diuresis can be achieved and, furthermore, that recovery is directly related to the occurrence of this diuresis. With advanced oliguric renal failure, diuretics are ineffective, and recovery can only occur when remission of the nephrotic syndrome allows for diuresis. On some occasions, renal failure may be irreversible during years of maintenance hemodialysis.[5] It must be presumed that persistent glomerular insufficiency such as this in the face of a minimal-change lesion is related to a mechanism that is dependent on the continuing glomerular leakage of protein and an inability to induce diuresis. However, since this form of acute renal failure occurs only rarely in MCNS despite the frequency of massive proteinuria, fluid retention, and relative oliguria, other mechanisms must be responsible that are initiated by the presence of nephrotic syndrome but are induced variably for reasons that at present are obscure.

Patients with MCNS who develop renal failure are often older than is usual for MCNS, and in fact the majority are over 50 years of age. Hypertension is common, as is microscopic hematuria. The nephrotic syndrome has been unusually severe for this group in that massive proteinuria is often associated with profound hypoalbuminemia under 1.5 g/dl. Further, in our own series, corticosteroid therapy failed to induce remission of the nephrotic syndrome in six of the 15 patients. This unusually high incidence of steroid resistance for MCNS[8] has also been observed by others reporting renal failure in MCNS. Finally, the rarity of acute renal failure in severe nephrotic states caused by other forms of glomerular disease is most striking and suggests that factors other than massive proteinuria and edema alone must be responsible for its occurrence almost exclusively in glomerular disease with minimal changes.

A hypothesis that is proposed to account for renal failure in MCNS must be consistent with the following: (1) a markedly reduced filtration fraction, (2) improvement in renal function coincident with induced diuresis, (3) further improvement in function with remission of nephrotic syndrome, (4) duration of renal failure prior to recovery as long as months, (5) renal failure only reversible if diuresis can be achieved, (6) renal failure persistent in face of extracorporeal ultrafiltration and elimination of edema in patients on dialysis, (7) recurrent renal failure with relapses of the nephrotic syndrome, (8) near exclusivity to nephrotic syndrome in minimal-change disease, in those with massive proteinuria and anasarca, yet still a rare occurrence, predominantly in the atypical older patients with MCNS.

It is generally held by most obsevers that renal failure in MCNS is attributable to hypovolemia resulting in renal vasoconstriction and hypoperfusion of the kidney with or without acute tubular necrosis (ATN). Rare cases of ATN have been reported, but more often the finding of a few necrotic or degenerating tubular cells has been seized as evidence of ATN for want of another anatomic diagnosis, even when the clinical course of the patients is clearly not compatible with this pathogenesis.

Several lines of evidence may be used to adduce that renal vasoconstriction consequent to decreased intravascular volume is not responsible for renal failure in MCNS. Measurements of glomerular filtration rate and renal plasma flow in our six patients demonstrated that filtration fraction was markedly reduced in all. This reduction stands in sharp contrast to the increase in filtration fraction that characterizes disorders such as hemorrhage or the hepatorenal syndrome, in which renal vasoconstriction and renal hypoperfusion are known to occur. Metcoff and Janeway described similar marked reductions in FF, attributable to a reduction in GFR out of proportion to that in renal plasma flow, in children with the nephrotic syndrome. Filtration fraction was below 0.10 in five of 18 children and increased toward normal following remission.[16] More recently, Dorhout Mees et al.[9] reported the finding of reduced creatinine and [^{51}Cr]EDTA clearances as well as depressed filtration fractions in a group of ten adult patients with minimal-change nephrotic syndrome who were selected for study because plasma volumes, measured with [^{131}I]serum albumin, were within normal limits. Following steroid-induced remission, GFR and filtration fraction increased in all; effective renal plasma flow was unchanged in three of seven patients and fell modestly in four.

Although plasma volumes were not measured in our patients, the improvement in GFR that occurred with diuresis in the face of continuing massive proteinuria argues against a causative role of hypovolemia since it is likely that plasma volume decreased rather than increased following induced diuresis. Although diuretic administration was accompanied by the infusion of salt-poor albumin in many of our patients, serum albumin concentration increased little (from a mean of 1.65 ± 0.11 to 2.31 ± 0.22 g/dl) in patients receiving salt-poor albumin; further, improvement in GFR was observed in response to diuretics without addition of albumin in six patients.

The arguments against renal vasoconstriction and ischemic ATN as the basis for renal failure in MCNS may be summarized as follows:

1. Blood volumes are in normal range.
2. Filtration fractions are inordinately reduced rather than elevated.
3. Recovery coincides with response to diuretics or remission of nephrotic syndrome.
4. When unresponsive to diuretics, renal failure may persist.
5. Renal failure may be irreversible.
6. Pattern of renal failure and its reversal with induced diuresis may be repetitive with relapses of nephrotic syndrome.
7. Renal morphology fails to support diagnosis of ATN.

What then may be proposed as a more likely mechanism for this unusual form of acute renal failure? As reported by a number of investigators, some reduction in GFR probably occurs in the majority of patients with MCNS, even though classically these individuals are characterized as nephrotics with "normal renal function, normal blood pressure, and no hematuria." Metcoff and Janeway found GFR reductions in 50% of a series of children with the nephrotic syndrome,[16] Hopper et al. in 60% of 31 patients,[17] and Dorhout Mees et al. in seven out of ten patients with MCNS. Robson et al. found an average reduction of 24% in inulin clearance of 11 children with MCNS.[9] The physiological basis for the reduction in GFR in MCNS is not known, but by analogy with studies in puromycin aminonucleoside (PAN)-induced nephrosis in the rat,[18, 19] a reduction in glomerular ultrafiltration coefficient could be responsible. In these studies, decreased glomerular capillary surface area was inferred from the finding of reduced fractional clearance of low-molecular-weight dextrans. Reversibility of reduced SNGFR in the PAN-induced nephrotic rat by saralasin raises the interesting possibility that the reduction in glomerular capillary surface area might be attributable to the vasoconstrictor effect of angiotensin II.

A frequent finding in the anatomic material obtained from patients with renal failure in MCNS has been the presence of dilated tubules, flattened epithelial cells, and proteinaceous casts containing degenerating tubular cells and debris. This has led to the proposal that tubular obstruction, which can be reversed by diuresis with or without remission of proteinuria, may be responsible for reduction of GFR in MCNS. Experimental evidence supporting a possible role of increased intratubular pressure may be derived from the studies of Kuroda et al.[20] in nephrotoxic serum nephritis-induced syndrome in the rat. Finding an increased pressure gradient between proximal and distal tubules, they postulated that proteinaceous fluid could be responsible for viscosity changes or cast formation in the thin limb, which would result in relative intratubular obstruction. Increased pressure in Bowman's space could then provide a mechanism for reduced net ultrafiltration pressure in MCNS.

Again, since high concentrations of protein in tubular fluid are common in severe nephrotic syndrome, the rare occurrence of more than minimal renal insufficiency requires the operation of an intermediate causative mechanism that is induced to a variable extent depending on individual predisposition. It may be postulated that increased intratubular pressure is responsible for the induction of vasoactive influences that adversely affect glomerular dynamics and filtering surface, as suggested by studies of experimental obstructive nephropathy that have demonstrated the operation of such interrelationships.[21]

Increased interstitial pressure resulting from renal edema may be still another cause of decreased net ultrafiltration pressure and reduced glomerular filtration rate in the nephrotic syndrome. Although direct evidence to support this hypothesis is lacking, the finding of marked reduction in filtration fraction by ourselves,[11] by Metcoff and Janeway,[16] and by Dorhout Mees et al.[9] and the observation that vigorous diuresis results in improvement in glomerular filtration would lend some support to this suggestion. In previous studies during osmotic diuresis in normal man and in patients with essential hypertension, we found an increase in intrarenal pressure as estimated by measurement of wedged renal vein pressure, which resulted in decreases in GFR and filtration fraction.[22] The decline in glomerular filtration rate could be accounted for in our studies by an increase in tubular hydrostatic pressure and consequent decrease in net filtration pressure. Renal plasma flow was unchanged or increased, with the result that filtration fraction fell significantly. Similarly, in the rat, massive osmotic diuresis results in a substantial increase in measured proximal tubular hydrostatic pressure, leading to decreased GFR and FF.[23] In the nephrotic syndrome, moderate reduction in filtration rate could be attributable to increased intrarenal pressure resulting from interstitial edema and would be reversible with diuresis.* However, the relatively infrequent occurrence of renal failure among the many patients with the nephrotic syndrome and massive fluid retention and the persistence of renal failure despite elimination of edema by ultrafiltration point up the inadequacy of the "interstitial pressure" hypothesis as the sole explanation for the varying degrees of renal insufficiency that can occur in MCNS.

The following hypothesis is tentatively proposed to account for the occurrence in MCNS of reversible renal insufficiency, which may range from minimal to severe:

1. The GFR and FF are generally reduced moderately in MCNS because of decreases in net ultrafiltration pressure and in ultrafiltration coefficient.
2. Reduction in net ultrafiltration pressure is attributable to increased proximal tubular pressure secondary to proteinaceous tubular fluid and to interstitial edema.
3. The ultrafiltration coefficient is reduced as a result of mesangial cell contraction, which may be induced by elevations in intratubular pressure through the release of vasoactive agents (possible role of angiotensin, prostaglandins).
4. Variability in the severity of GFR depression reflects individual differences in the magnitude of this vasoactive response.
5. In some instances, especially the elderly with hypertension, oliguric renal failure supervenes as a consequence of drastic alterations in the determinants of glomerular filtration resulting from exaggerated vasoactive influences.
6. Diuresis, either diuretic-induced or resulting from remission of the primary glomerular disease, can reverse reductions in GFR by washout of proteinaceous tubular fluid, by reduction in interstitial pressure, and by consequent abrogation of the vasoactive response.

---

*Based on our earlier measurements of WRVP,[22] glomerular ultrafiltration pressure (P_{UF}) was estimated to be 12.5 mm Hg in normal man. Assuming that the observed decrease in GFR in MCNS is attributable solely to an increase in hydrostatic pressure in Bowman's space (i.e., that K_f is unchanged) and allowing for the decrease in $\bar{\pi}$ resulting from decreased serum albumin concentration and decreased filtration fraction, we can estimate that an increase of P_T to 47 mm Hg would be required to account for an 80% reduction in GFR. This value was attained during osmotic diuresis in normal subjects.[22] If the observed 40% decrease in renal blood flow reflects increased afferent arteriolar resistance, glomerular hydrostatic pressure would be correspondingly decreased, and even lesser increases in tubular hydrostatic pressure would suffice to account for the decrease in GFR.

7. In the case of oliguric renal failure, diuresis cannot be induced. Renal failure persists on dialysis despite elimination of edema by ultrafiltration; presumably, increased intratubular pressure caused by casts and proteinaceous fluid continues to provoke the vasoactive response.

8. Recovery of function may still occur after a protracted period of renal failure if nephrotic syndrome ultimately remits, allowing washout of proteinaceous fluid and reversal of vasoactive influences on the glomerular capillary filtering bed.

An explanation for the great variability in the degree of GFR reduction in MCNS and the predisposition of the most severe and prolonged forms of renal failure to occur in certain few individuals, particularly the elderly with hypertension, defies speculation. Equally obscure is the reason for the rarity of acute renal failure in other glomerular diseases that may be associated with severe nephrotic syndrome. The precise nature of the vasoactive mechanisms that mediate this form of glomerular failure, reversible by diuresis whether or not accompanied by remission of proteinuria, remains to be explored.

REFERENCES

1. Folli G, Pollak VE, Reid RTW, et al: Electronmicroscopic studies of reversible glomerular lesions in the adult nephrotic syndrome. *Ann Intern Med* 49:775-795, 1958
2. Chamberlain MJ, Pringle A, Wrong OM: Oliguric renal failure in the nephrotic syndrome with minimal glomerular pathology. *J Med* 35:215-235, 1966
3. Conolly ME, Wrong OM, Jones NF: Reversible renal failure in idiopathic nephrotic syndrome with minimal glomerular pathology. *Quart J Med* 35:215-235, 1966
4. Cameron JS, Turner DR, Ogg CS, et al: The nephrotic syndrome in adults with 'minimal change' glomerular lesions. *Quart J Med* 43:461-488, 1974
5. Raij L, Keane WF, Leonard A, et al: Irreversible acute renal failure in idiopathic nephrotic syndrome. *Am J Med* 61:207-214, 1976
6. Case Records of the Massachusetts General Hospital. *N Engl J Med* 299:136-145, 1978
7. Holdsworth DR, Stephenson P, Dowling JP, et al: Reversible acute renal failure in the nephrotic syndrome with minimal glomerular pathology. *Med J Aust* 2:532-533, 1977
8. Stephens VJ, Yates APB, Lechler RI, et al: Reversible uraemia in normotensive nephrotic syndrome. *Br Med J* 2:705-706, 1979
9. Dorhout Mees EJ, Roos JC, Boer P, et al: Observation on edema formation in the nephrotic syndrome and adults with minimal lesions. *Am J Med* 67:378-384, 1979
10. Hulter HN, Bonner EL Jr: Lipoid nephrosis appearing as acute oliguric renal failure. *Arch Intern Med* 140:403-405, 1980
11. Lowenstein J, Schacht RG, Baldwin DS: Renal failure in minimal change nephrotic syndrome. *Am J Med* 70:227-233, 1981
12. Esparza AR, Kahn SI, Garella S, et al: Spectrum of acute renal failure in nephrotic syndrome with minimal (or minor) glomerular lesions. *Lab Invest* 45:510-521, 1981

13. Case Records of the Massachusetts General Hospital. *N Engl J Med* 306:221-231, 1982
14. Sjoberg RJ, McMillan VM, Bartram LS, et al: Renal failure with minimal change nephrotic syndrome: Reversal with hemodialysis. *Clin Nephrol* 20:98-100, 1983
15. McCluskey RT, Vassalli P, Gallo GR, et al: An immunofluorescent study of pathogenetic mechanisms in glomerular diseases. *N Engl J Med* 274:695-701, 1966
16. Metcoff J, Janeway CA: Studies on the pathogenesis of nephrotic edema. *Pediatrics* 58:640-685, 1961
17. Hopper J, Ryan P, Lee JC: Lipoid nephrosis in 31 adult patients. *Medicine* 49:321-341, 1970
18. Bohrer MP, Baylis C, Robertson CR, et al: Mechanisms of the puromycin-induced defects in the transglomerular passage of water and macromolecules. *J Clin Invest* 60:152-161, 1977
19. Ichikawa I, Rennke HG, Hoyer JR, et al: Role for intrarenal mechanisms in the impaired salt excretion of experimental nephrotic syndrome. *J Clin Invest* 71:91-102, 1983
20. Kuroda S, Aynedjian HS, Bank N: A micropuncture study of renal sodium retention in nephrotic syndrome in rats: Evidence for increased resistance to tubular fluid flow. *Kidney Int* 16:561-571, 1979
21. Klahr S: Nephrology forum: Pathophysiology of obstructive uropathy. *Kidney Int* 23:414-426, 1983
22. Lowenstein J, Beranbaum ER, Chasis H, et al: Intrarenal pressure and exaggerated natriuresis in essential hypertension. *Clin Sci* 38:359-374, 1970
23. Koch KM, Dume W, Krause HH, et al: Intratubulärer Druck glomerularer Capillardruck and glomerulum Filtrat während Mannet-Diurese. *Pfluegers Arch* 295:72-29, 1967

8

Proteinuria in Diabetic Renal Allograft Recipients

JAMES M. LUCIANO, ARAM V. MANOUKIAN,
KHALID M. H. BUTT, AND ELI A. FRIEDMAN

INTRODUCTION

Recipients of renal allografts commonly manifest proteinuria for months to years after transplantation,[1,2] apparently without increased mortality compared to nonproteinuric recipients. Posttransplant proteinuria has been attributed to chronic allograft rejection[1-3] or recurrent glomerulonephritis[4,5]; histological studies of renal allografts demonstrate both processes within months after transplantation.[1,6] Proteinuria is a constant concomitant finding in diabetic nephropathy and is correlated with duration of diabetes. Approximately 10% to 30% of all diabetics develop proteinuria[7] because of glomerular structural injury and increased permeability resulting from diabetic nephropathy.[8,9] Glomerulosclerosis is found in 90% of type I diabetics of longer than 10 years' duration.[10] Progressive nephropathy is likely once constant proteinuria develops; 80% of proteinuric diabetics die within 11 years of its discovery, and about half of these deaths are from renal failure.[7] On average, death occurs 7 years following the onset of persistent proteinuria.

During the early 1980s, the proportion of kidney transplant recipients who are diabetic increased to 25%,[11] and determination of the significance of posttransplant proteinuria has become essential to defining the natural history of the nephropathy that recurs in kidneys obtained from nondiabetics and transplanted into diabetics. It is known that diabetic nephropathy recurs within 2 to 3 years in the majority of kidneys obtained from nondiabetic donors and transplanted into diabetic

JAMES M. LUCIANO, ARAM V. MANOUKIAN, KHALID M. H. BUTT, AND ELI A. FRIEDMAN • Departments of Medicine and Surgery, Downstate Medical Center, Brooklyn, New York 11203.

recipients.[11] The current investigation was conducted to ascertain whether proteinuria in diabetic kidney recipients differs in prevalence or severity from that in nondiabetic recipients.

PATIENTS AND METHODS

Patient Selection

Stable renal transplant recipients were studied after obtaining their informed consent. Patients were selected to participate in this study by requesting their cooperation at routine clinic visits or during hospitalizations for causes other than rejection or failure of their renal graft from any cause. There were 21 diabetic and nondiabetic consecutive and available adult recipients who provided urine and blood samples. Repeat blood and urine studies were performed in 15 diabetics and 22 nondiabetics. All but three diabetic recipients were studied as outpatients. Patients were excluded from study if hospitalized for (1) continued observation immediately post-transplant (usually 2 to 3 weeks), (2) diagnosis and treatment of an acute rejection episode, or (3) during the course of any febrile illness.

Diabetic Patients

Diabetes mellitus was established as a diagnosis in the medical record of each patient counted as diabetic. Of 21 diabetic recipients, a subset of 15 patients who were diabetic prior to kidney transplantation comprised the group of "pretransplant diabetics." The remaining six patients among the 21 diabetic recipients were first noted to be diabetic after transplantation and constituted the group of "posttransplant diabetics." All pre- and posttransplant diabetics required insulin prior to and during the study period. Of the 15 pretransplant diabetics, three had previously been maintained on oral hypoglycemic drugs and were probably type II diabetics. The native kidneys of four pretransplant diabetic recipients had been biopsied, and three exhibited diabetic glomerulosclerosis; the fourth biopsy yielded insufficient tissue for a diagnosis.

Nondiabetic Patients

The renal diagnosis was taken from the medical record. A percutaneous renal biopsy of the native kidneys of nine of 26 nondiabetics had been performed prior to transplantation, from which the following diagnoses were made: focal glomerular sclerosis (3), membranoproliferative glomerulonephritis (2), systemic lupus erythematosus (1), and rapidly progressive glomerulonephritis (1). An inconclusive diagnosis was made in two biopsies. Clinical diagnoses in five additional nondiabetic patients were hereditary nephritis, Lawrence Moon–Biedl syndrome, polyarteritis nodosa, and polycystic kidney disease (2). Biopsy reports were unavailable or biopsies were not performed for remaining patients.

Transplant Regimen

The immunosuppressive regimen for diabetic and nondiabetic patients consisted of initial doses of azathioprine (2 mg/kg) and prednisone (1.5 mg/kg), which were then progressively reduced. A "rejection episode" was defined as a hospital admission prior to the onset of the present study necessitated by allograft rejection during which the patient was treated for rejection. Rejection episodes had been treated by intravenous doses of methylprednisolone (120 to 1000 mg for 2 to 10 days) and/or antithymocyte globulin (15 mg/kg intravenously for 7 to 14 days). Cyclosporin A was continued in one diabetic patient after having been begun elsewhere (Pittsburgh, Dr. T. Starzl). All but one nondiabetic patient retained their native kidneys post-transplant.

Laboratory Methods

Sampling Protocol. Hospitalized patients were studied on the transplant ward. Ambulatory patients brought 24h urine collections to an outpatient clinic, at which time a clean-catch urine specimen was collected for urinalysis and routine culture. Venous blood was drawn from an antecubital vein for determination of serum creatinine, blood urea nitrogen, and serum glucose by standard techniques using the SMA 6/60 Technicon Autoanalyser (Tarrytown, NY). The hemoglobin and hematocrit were determined using an electronic counter, the Coulter S Plus (Hialeah, FL). Glycosylated hemoglobin concentration was determined at a commercial laboratory by the method of Trivelli et al.[13] (Metpath, Teterboro and Hackensack, NJ). Total serum protein was determined by standard methods, and cellulose acetate protein electrophoresis was quantitated with a densitometer.

Collection and Storage of 24-h Urine. Total daily urine specimens were collected in plastic jugs or, on some occasions, in clean and dry glass jars from the patient's home. Patients were asked to refrigerate their specimens if possible. No preservative was added. On receipt, the total urine volume was measured, and two 50-ml aliquots were frozen at -65°C in polystyrene centrifuge tubes. Urine specimens were kept frozen until a β_2-microglobulin assay was performed; once thawed, they were stored at 0–4°C until urinary creatinine, total protein, and protein electrophoresis were quantified.

Measurement and Characterization of Urinary Protein. Total urinary protein was determined by a sulfosalicylic acid technique.[14] To fractionate urinary proteins, a 20-ml aliquot of the 24-h urine collection was concentrated 100 times using an Amicon microfilter prior to cellulose acetate electrophoresis. The fractions were then quantitated using a densitometer that detected proteins in concentrations greater than 40 to 50mg/liter. Both analyses were performed at the previously referenced commercial laboratory. The urinary β_2-microglobulin concentration was determined by radioimmunoassay using the Phadebas β_2-Microtest Kit (Pharmacia, Inc., Piscataway, NJ).[15]

Measurement of Urinary Creatinine. Creatinine concentration in urine was determined by an alkaline picrate method[15] performed on the Centrifi-Chem System 500 (Union Carbide, Rye, NY).

Statistical Analysis

Because frequency distributions of the urinary total protein determinations were highly skewed, nonparametric statistics were used to analyze the data obtained. If patients were tested on two occasions, the values of each laboratory test were averaged. Group comparisons were made using the normal approximation to the Wilcoxon Rank-Sum Test.[17] The Spearman Rank Correlation Coefficient was calculated to determine associations between the amount of total urinary protein and other variables.[18] Differences and associations were defined as significant at the 0.05 level (i.e., $P < 0.05$).

RESULTS

Details of the patient groups studied, nondiabetic and pretransplant and posttransplant diabetic recipients, are given in Table I. Also listed in Table I are key urinary, hematologic, and biochemical data in the three patient groups. Patients in both diabetic groups were older (by a mean of 7 years for pretransplant diabetics and a mean of 15 years for posttransplant diabetics) than the nondiabetic recipients. Both groups of dia-

Table I. Characteristics of Nondiabetic, Pretransplant Diabetic,
and Posttransplant Diabetic Recipients (Mean ± S.D.)

	Nondiabetics	Pretransplant diabetics	Posttransplant diabetics
Number of subjects	26	15	6
Males	13	12	3
Females	13	3	3
Age	30 ± 11.8	37 ± 9.2[a]	45 ± 10.1[b]
	(10–53)	(31–57)	(32–58)
Time post-transplant	27 ± 21.7	18 ± 23.4	6 ± 20.2[c]
(mos)	(1–75)	(1–82)	(2–54)
No. related donors	8	7	0
No. previous grafts	7	2	1
No. rejection episodes	26[d]	16	7
Mean blood pressure	92 ± 12.8	98 ± 10.0[e]	104 ± 17.2[f]
(mm Hg)[g]	(70–113)	(80–112)	(76–116)
Hemoglobin A_1C (%)	6.4 ± 1.4	11.0 ± 1.9	10.7 ± 3.0
(nl: 4.4–8.2%)	(3.2–9.1)	(6.3–12.5)	(6.3–14.5)
Blood urea nitrogen	24 ± 19.6	30 ± 18.5	29 ± 24.8
(nl: 10–20 mg/dl)	(15–96)	(20–66)	(16–82)
Serum creatinine	1.4 ± 1.1	1.6 ± 0.8	1.7 ± 0.5
(nl: 0.4–1.5 mg/dl)	(0.7–6.3)	(1.0–3.8)	(1.1–2.5)
Hematocrit (%)	41.0 ± 8.0	40.5 ± 7.0	41.8 ± 6.3
	(20.7–51.7)	(26.0–47.2)	(32.6–51.7)
Creatinine clearance	63.2 ± 35.7	67.3 ± 28.4	88.0 ± 75.9
(ml/min)	(8.2–160.0)	(11.8–???.?)	(24.1–160.3)
Duration of diabetes		21 ± 8.0 yr	2 ± 2.0 mo
		(6–33 yr)	(1–5 mo)

[a]$P < 0.02$ compared with the nondiabetic group.
[b]$P < 0.025$ compared with the nondiabetic group.
[c]$P < 0.0002$ compared with the nondiabetic group.
[d]Medical record unavailable for two nondiabetic patients.
[e]Blood pressures obtained for 12 of 15 patients in this group.
[f]Blood pressures obtained for five of six patients in this group.
[g]Mean blood pressure = systolic − (systolic − diastolic/3).

betics had higher random serum glucose and glycosylated hemoglobin values than the controls. Of 20 diabetics tested, seven had a normal level of glycosylated hemoglobin; two nondiabetics, both 13-year-old girls, had abnormally high values despite having normal serum glucose levels. Posttransplant diabetics produced significantly ($p < 0.01$) more urine (mean of 3152 ml/day) than did the nondiabetics (mean of 2308 ml/day). Nondiabetic recipients had been transplanted earlier (27 months) than either diabetic group, but this difference was only of statistical significance for the posttransplant diabetics. In contrast to the nondiabetic and posttransplant diabetic groups, the pretransplant diabetic group was comprised mostly of male patients.

Urinary infections were uncommon in all groups. Only two patients had bacteriuria. One pretransplant diabetic patient had greater than 100,000 colonies/ml of *Citrobacter diversus* on two occasions with pyuria noted in one sample. A second pretransplant diabetic had greater than 100,000 colonies/ml of *Candida albicans* in one sample accompanied by pyuria, hematuria, and many budding yeast. Two nondiabetic recipients and two pretransplant diabetics had greater than five white blood cells per high-power field on routine urinalysis in the presence of negative urine cultures.

The pretransplant diabetics had been diabetic for a mean of 21 years; the posttransplant diabetics developed diabetes between 1 and 6 months prior to evaluation (a range of 1 to 5 months after transplantation).

Serum Protein Analysis

Serum protein concentrations in the three groups are given in Table II. Total serum protein concentrations and the levels of albumin, α-globulins 1 and 2, β-globulin, and γ-globulin were similar among all three groups. Mean albumin concentrations in the three groups ranged from 4.0 g/dl (posttransplant diabetics) to 4.3 g/dl (nondiabetics).

Urinary Protein Analysis

Daily urinary protein excretion was similar in the three groups (Table III). Although pretransplant and posttransplant diabetic groups had higher median levels of total urinary protein and β_2-microglobulin excretion than did nondiabetics, the differences were not significant. Of 47 patients tested, only three, all of whom were nondiabetics, had daily protein excretion below 130 mg. The majority of nondiabetic and pretransplant diabetic recipients excreted between 0.14 and 1.00 g of protein per 24 h. Nephrotic-range proteinuria was rare. Only three of 47 patients (6.4%), none of whom was a pretransplant diabetic, excreted more than 3.5 g/day.

β_2-microglobulin excretion was similar in diabetic and nondiabetic groups. The median level of urinary β_2-microglobulin was highest in posttransplant diabetics, but this difference was not significant. We did not measure β_2-microglobulin excretion in normal, healthy patients without renal allografts. Median levels of β_2-microglobulin excretion in the three groups studied, however, were above normal according to the standardized assay and comprised from 1% to 2% of total protein excre-

Table II. Serum Protein Concentration (gm/dl) in Nondiabetic, Pretransplant
Diabetic and Posttransplant Diabetic Recipients

	Nondiabetics	Pretransplant Diabetics	Posttransplant Diabetics
Number of subjects	25	15	6
Total protein	7.3 ± 0.7	7.1 ± 0.7	7.4 ± 0.2
(nl: 6.20–8.30)	(5.5–9.1)	(5.5–7.7)	(7.0–8.1)
Albumin	4.3 ± 0.52	4.2 ± 0.36	4.0 ± 0.16
(nl: 3.10–5.00)	(3.2–4.8)	(2.9–4.9)	(3.9–4.2)
$\alpha 1$	0.16 ± 0.04	0.16 ± 0.07	0.19 ± 0.08
(nl: 0.15–0.40)	(0.10–0.24)	(0.06–0.29)	(0.13–0.36)
$\alpha 2$	0.59 ± 0.16	0.70 ± 1.4	0.62 ± 0.19
(nl: 0.50–1.00)	(0.29–1.01)	(0.56–1.23)	(0.54–0.98)
β	0.70 ± 0.16	0.75 ± 0.18	0.77 ± 0.15
(nl: 0.60–1.20)	(0.43–1.13)	(0.55–1.20)	(0.45–0.86)
γ	11.21 ± 0.41	1.23 ± 09.29	1.24 ± 0.67
(nl: 0.60–1.60)	(0.53–2.47)	(0.42–1.55)	(0.96–2.79)

tion for diabetic and nondiabetic groups, respectively. Fractional components of urinary immunoglobulins were similar in the three groups.

There was no significant correlation between urinary protein excretion and age, the interval between transplantation and evaluation, random serum glucose, glycosylated hemoglobin value, creatinine clearance, or urine volume (Table IV). In each group, patients with renal allografts

Table III. Urinary Protein Excretion in Nondiabetic, Pretransplant
Diabetic and Posttransplant Diabetic Recipients (g/24h)

	Nondiabetics	Pretransplant Diabetics	Posttransplant Diabetics
Number of subjects	26	15	6
Protein excretion			
0.00–0.13	3	0	0
0.14–1.00	17	12	0
1.01–2.00	3	1	2
2.01–3.49	1	2	1
>3.50	2	0	1
Total protein*	0.35 ± 1.82	0.52 ± 0.75	1.37 ± 1.41
(range)[a]	(0.09–8.52)	(0.25–2.56)	(0.42–3.92)
$\beta 2$-Microglobulin	0.010 ± 0.013^{c}	0.006 ± 0.028	0.013 ± 0.40
(range)[b]	(0.00–0.044)	(0.00–0.095)	(0.00–0.106)

[a]Total protein normal range: 0.00–0.13 μg/24h.
[b]$\beta 2$-microglobulin normal range reported by Pharmacia Diagnostics: 30–370 μg/24h.
[c]Values obtained for 25 of the 26 patients in this group.

Table IV. Urinary Protein Electrophoresis in Nondiabetic,
Pretransplant Diabetic and Posttransplant Diabetic Recipients

	Nondiabetics	Pretransplant Diabetics	Posttransplant Diabetics
Number of subjects	26	15	6
Normal pattern	20	12	4
Abnormal pattern[a]	6	3	2
Albumin	76 ± 8.2	66 ± 9.0	80 ± 2.8
α-Globulins	4 ± 2.1	6 ± 3.5	3 ± 2.5
β-Globulins	8 ± 3.0	7 ± 2.9	8 ± 2.5
γ-Globulins	10 ± 3.9	13 ± 4.4	10 ± 3.2

[a]For each constituent of the abnormal pattern defined, the median percentage of the total urine protein is presented; for this reason, values, when summed, may not equal 100%.

of cadaveric origin and those with grafts from living related donors had similar amounts of proteinuria; the number of rejection episodes and the number of histocompatibility antigens matched were unrelated to the amount of proteinuria. Mean blood pressure and β_2-microglobulin excretion were significantly correlated with total urinary protein level in posttransplant diabetic and nondiabetic groups, respectively; these variables were not correlated with proteinuria in any of the other groups. The concentration of serum protein was inversely related to the amount of proteinuria for the nondiabetic group alone.

DISCUSSION

Proteinuria following renal allografting is usual in the first week and consists of both glomerular (high-molecular-weight) and tubular (low-molecular-weight) proteins.[19,20] In succeeding weeks of stable allograft function, proteinuria typically lessens, becomes tubular in character, and may disappear by the end of the first year.[19] Immediate posttransplant proteinuria has been attributed to renal ischemia and appears unrelated to the presence or absence of the patient's original diseased kidneys.[21] Months to years after transplantation, however, despite continued allograft function, persistent proteinuria may recur[1-3,22] because of either chronic rejection or recurrent glomerulonephritis.[4,5] The amount of proteinuria in one report[1] of long-term renal transplant recipients was associated with the number and severity of acute rejection episodes and the degree of histocompatibility between donor and recipient. In our study, correlation between the number of rejection episodes and the amount of proteinuria was less than significant for diabetics and nondiabetics.

The present study demonstrates that diabetic and nondiabetic long-term renal transplant recipients excrete similar amounts of urinary protein. In addition, it confirms the observation that most long-term renal allograft recipients have significant proteinuria. All diabetic recipients excreted more than 0.13 g/day of urinary protein, and 88% of nondiabetics had proteinuria of this magnitude. We were surprised to find that only three of 47 recipients had nephrotic-range proteinuria, only one of whom was diabetic. For comparison, Harlan et al.[1] reported that 79% of long-term allograft recipients had proteinuria and that 24% of their patients had nephrotic-range proteinuria. Westberg et al.[3] reported the average total urinary protein concentration of 16 long-term recipients as 1.1 g/day. A higher prevalence (30%) of heavy proteinuria was also note by Cheigh et al.[2]

Cellulose acetate electrophoresis of urine proteins revealed that most patients, whether diabetic or nondiabetic, exhibited a normal pattern. This form of electrophoresis, however, is not sufficiently sensitive to differentiate among various types of urinary protein if proteinuria is not heavy—only albumin is detectable when total excretion is low. Albumin comprises about 40% of total urinary protein in healthy individuals.[22] Urinary protein excretion in long-term recipients analyzed by an immunoprecipitin reaction[22] shows a poorly selective mixed glomerulotubular pattern. The proteinuria of diabetic nephropathy is also nonselective[23] but, in contrast to proteinuria in long-term renal allograft recipients, does not contain an increased concentration of β_2-microglobulin, a tubular protein.

In each of our study groups, the level of β_2-microglobulin was between 20 and 90 times higher than that reported by Hemmingsen et al.[22] We are unable to distinguish between increased synthesis and decreased reabsorption to account for this finding. Radioimmunoassay, a more sensitive method for identifying urinary proteins, might clarify the origin of the "excess" β_2-microglobulin.

An association has previously been reported between urinary protein excretion and elevated blood pressure.[24,25] Antihypertensive therapy reduces albuminuria in hypertensive diabetic patients.[26,27] In the present study, proteinuria and mean blood pressure were significantly correlated in six patients who developed diabetes after transplantation, but not in the other diabetics or nondiabetics. Harlan et al.[1] found a higher mean blood pressure in long-term renal allograft recipients excreting more than 3 g/day than in allograft recipients with lesser proteinuria. It is unclear, however, how many of these patients were diabetic.

Sustained hyperglycemia is associated with proteinuria.[28] Viberti et al.[29] reported that urinary albumin excretion was significantly reduced when blood glucose was strictly controlled by insulin infusion in seven

clinically nonproteinuric diabetics. Establishment of sustained euglyce-
mia by continuous subcutaneous insulin infusion in proteinuric type I
diabetics apparently does not reduce proteinuria.[30] Stephen et al., on
the other hand, have found that a regimen in which insulin is administered by an intraperitoneal device to proteinuric type I diabetics
does reduce the quantity of protein leakage.[31] A key issue in the
management of diabetes is the degree to which glucose regulation should
be attempted in the hope of preventing (reversing) microvascular complications of retinopathy and glomerulopathy.[32] Mauer et al.[12] found
that ten of 12 diabetic renal allograft recipients had recurrent diabetic
nephropathy in the transplant after 2 or more years, but only three of
these patients had histological evidence of chronic rejection. More recently, Mauer et al. reported recurrence of mesangial and glomerular
basement membrane changes typical of diabetic nephropathy in normal
living related and cadaver kidneys transplanted into diabetic patients after 2 years.[33] Approximately a third of our diabetics had had their grafts
for 2 years or more, but they could not be distinguished from their nondiabetic counterparts by creatinine clearance or the amount of proteinuria.

The amount of proteinuria in diabetic and nondiabetic patients in our
study did not correlate with either a random blood glucose level or the
level of glycosylated hemoglobin. The observation that albuminuria may
be reduced in clinically nonproteinuric diabetics by strict glucose control
suggests that functional rather than morphological factors were
reversed.[29] Whether the effort demanded of patient and physician to
normalize blood glucose levels in diabetic kidney transplant recipients
will prevent or minimize recurrence of diabetic glomerulosclerosis or alter
severity of chronic allograft rejection is undetermined. Assessment of the
course of proteinuric diabetic kidney transplant recipients subjected to
strict versus usual control will be required to resolve this debate.

We were impressed with the low rate of urinary infection in diabetic
and nondiabetic transplant recipients. It is remarkable that neither past
instrumentation (all had had urethral catheters for days), immunosuppression, nor previous bladder surgery induced persistent bacteriuria in
more than 6.4% of recipients.

ACKNOWLEDGMENTS. We are indebted to Robert Galonsky, Mildred
Hirshman, Veronica Henry, Benjamin Richardson, and Jack Deutsch for
technical support, Dr. Rober DeCreasce for providing the radioimmunoassay kits, Sondra Hirsch, R.N., and Pamela Brandon, R.N., for
their help in arranging for facilities, and Monica Beyer for continued en-
couragement.

REFERENCES

1. Harlan WR, Holden KR, Williams GN, et al: Proteinuria and nephrotic syndrome associated with chronic rejection of kidney transplants. *N Engl J Med* 277:767-776, 1967
2. Cheigh JS, Stenzel KH, Susin M, et al: Kidney transplant nephrotic syndrome. *Am J Med* 57:730-740, 1974
3. Westberg G., Bergentz S., Hood B.: Renal function and protein excretion in kidney transplants functioning for 6 to 26 months. *Scand J Urol Nephrol* 2:53-57, 1968
4. Hamburger J, Crosnier J., Dormont J.: Observations in patients with a well-tolerated homotransplant kidney. *Ann NY Acad Sci* 120:558-556, 1964
5. Dixon FJ, McPhail J, Lerner R: The contribution of kidney transplantation to the study of glomerulonephritis—the recurrence of glomerulonephritis in renal transplants. *Transplant Proc* 1:194-196, 1969
6. Hulme B, Anders GA, Porter KA, et al: Human renal transplants IV. Glomerular ultrastructure, macromolecular permeability and hemodynamics. *Lab Invest* 26:2-10, 1972
7. Knowles HL: Magnitude of the renal failiure problem in diabetes. *Kidney Int [Suppl. 1]* 6:2-7, 1974
8. Parving H-H: Increased microvascular permeabilty to plasma proteins in short and long term juvenile diabetes. *Diabetes [Supp. 2]* 25:884-889, 1976
9. Williamson JR, Kilo C: Current status of capillary basement membrane disease in diabetes mellitus. *Diabetes* 26:65-73, 1977
10. Mauer SM, Steffes MW, Goetz FC, et al: Diabetic nephropathy. A perspective. *Diabetes* 32:S52-S55, 1983
11. Friedman EA: Is diabetic nephropathy preventable? A billion dollar question. *Diabetic Nephropathy* 1:1, 1982
12. Mauer SM, Barbosa J, Vernier R, et al: Development of diabetic vascular lesions in normal kidneys transplanted into patients with diabetes mellitus. *N Engl J Med* 295:916-920, 1976
13. Trivelli L, Ranney HM, Lai HT: Hemoglobin components in patients with diabetes mellitus. *N Engl J Med* 284:353-357, 1971
14. Henry RJ, Cannon DC, Winkelman JW: *Clinical Chemistry: Principles and Technics*, ed 2. Hagerstown, Harper & Row, 1974, pp 434-435
15. Evrin PE, Petersen PA, Wide L, et al: Radioimmunoassay of β_2-microglobulin in human biological fluids. *Scand J Clin Lab Invest* 28:439-443, 1971
16. Henry RJ, Cannon DC, Winkelman JW: *Clinical Chemistry Principles and Technics*, ed 2. Hagerstwon, Harper & Row, 1974, pp 552-553
17. Leach C: *Introduction to Statistics: A Nonparametric Approach for the Social Sciences*. Chichester, John Wiley & Sons, 1979, pp 58-78
18. Siegel S: *Nonparametric Statistics for the Behavioral Sciences*. New York, McGraw-Hill, 1959, pp 206-213
19. Manuel Y, Poli S, Bernhardt P, et al: Proteinuria in human renal allografts. *Helv Med Acta* 35:3-19, 1969
20. Sethi K, First MR, Pesce AJ, et al: Proteinuria following renal transplantation. *Nephron* 18:49-59, 1977
21. Debray-Sachs M: Study of proteinuria after kidney transplantation with long-term survival, Manuel Y, Revillard JP, Betuel H (eds): *Proteins in Normal and Pathological Urine*. Baltimore, University Park Press, 1970, pp 270-280
22. Hemmingsen L, Jensen H, Skaarup P: The urinary excretion of ten plasma proteins in long-term renal transplant patients. *Acta Med Scand* 199:311-316, 1976

23. Jones RH, Marshall W, Myers R, et al: The proteinuria of diabetic nephropathy. *Clin Chim Acta* 108:375–383, 1980
24. Parving H-H, Jensen H, Mogensen CE, et al: Increased urinary albumin excretion in benign essential hypertension. *Lancet* 1:1190–1192, 1974
25. Pedersen E, Mogenson C: Effect of antihypertensive treatment of urinary albumin excretion, glomerular filtration rate, and renal plasma flow in patient with essential hypertension. *Scand J Clin Lab Invest* 36:231–237, 1976
26. Parving H-H, Andersen AR, Smidt V, et al: Reduced albuminuria during early and aggressive antihypertensive treatment of insulin-dependent diabetic patients with diabetic nephropathy. *Diabetes Care* 4:459–463, 1981
27. Mogensen CE: Progression of nephropathy in long-term diabetes with proteinuria and effect of initial antihypertensive treatment. *Scand J Clin Lab Invest* 36:383–388, 1976
28. Parving H-H: Microvascular permeability to plasma proteins in hypertension and diabetes mellitus in man—on the pathogenesis of hypertensive and diabetic neuroangiopathy. *Dan Med Bull* 22:217–233, 1975
29. Viberti GC, Pickup J, Jarrett RJ, et al: Effect of control of blood glucose on urinary excretion of albumin and β_2-microglobulin in insulin-dependent diabetes. *N Engl J Med* 300:638–641, 1979
30. Viberti GC, Bilous RW, Mackintosh D, et al: Monitoring glomerular function in diabetic nephropathy. A prospective study. *Am J Med* 74:256–264, 1983
31. Stephern RL, Maddock RK, Kablitz C, et al: Stabilization and improvement of renal function in diabetic nephropathy. *Diabetic Nephropathy* 1:8–13, 1982
32. Friedman EA: Diabetic nephropathy: Strategies in prevention and management. *Kidney Int* 21:780–791, 1982
33. Mauer SM, Steffes MW, Connett J, et al: The development of lesions in the glomerular basement membrane and mesangium after transplantation of normal kidneys to diabetic patients. *Diabetes* 32:948–952, 1983

9

Proteinuria following Renal Transplantation

KURT H. STENZEL, JHOONG S. CHEIGH,
JANET MOURADIAN, JOHN WANG, AND ILENE MILLER

INTRODUCTION

As more and more patients receive renal transplants, diseases of transplanted kidneys and problems related to immunosuppression will be more and more frequently encountered by nephrologists. At our center alone, we will soon complete over 1000 kidney transplant procedures with an experience that spans 20 years. Proteinuria, a common sign of kidney disease, is often found following transplantation, and when it occurs, it requires careful and detailed evaluation. Mechanisms responsible for posttransplant proteinuria are varied, often multifactorial, and must be ascertained for each patient. Lesions associated with proteinuria may result from rejection, infection, obstruction, recurrent disease, or *de novo* glomerulonephritis or interstitial nephritis. In addition, there is growing concern about the effects of renal hyperperfusion in patients with decreased renal mass and the possible development of nephropathy secondary to this increased plasma flow, both in recipients and in donors of transplanted kidneys.[1] Drug-induced renal disease may become an increasingly severe problem with more widespread use of the nephrotoxic immunosuppressant cyclosporin in kidney transplant recipients.

In this chapter, we review several aspects of posttransplant proteinuria, including the incidence and clinical spectrum of posttransplant nephrotic syndrome and the relationship between transplant biopsy findings and the clinical course in nephrotic patients, the incidence and interpretation of focal segmental glomerulosclerosis in transplant recipients,

KURT H. STENZEL, JHOONG S. CHEIGH, JANET MOURADIAN, JOHN WANG, AND ILENE MILLER • Rogosin Kidney Center, Departments of Medicine, Biochemistry, and Pathology, The New York Hospital–Cornell Medical Center, New York, New York 10021.

and the significance of proteinuria and hypertension in patients with well-functioning grafts many years after transplant, and address the problems of hypertension, proteinuria, and decreasing renal function in kidney transplant donors.

The overall posttransplant course depends on many variables including pretransplant blood transfusions, type of donor, HLA incompatibilities, and type of immunosuppression used. The patients whom we discuss received imuran and prednisone as the sole immunosuppressant therapy, and these drugs were used in relatively low doses. Some of the patients also received a human γ-globulin preparation that has an effect on prolonging graft survival but does not suppress the immune response, nor does it have a direct nephrotoxic effect. The immunosuppressive regimen has previously been outlined in detail.[2] In addition, immunologic responsiveness is closely monitored, and the data obtained are used as a guide to individualize the dose of the immunosuppressive agents.[3] Using these methods, we have attained a posttransplant survival of over 90% at 3 years and markedly decreased the incidence of infections common to immunosuppressed patients.[4]

POSTTRANSPLANT NEPHROTIC SYNDROME

Proteinuria frequently occurs in the immediate posttransplant period and has little or no significance for the eventual outcome of the transplant.[5,6] It may also occur transiently during acute rejection episodes.[6] A more serious problem is the development of persistent proteinuria and the nephrotic syndrome in patients with functioning grafts. In a study of 599 renal allografts at our center,[7] 54 developed the nephrotic syndrome, defined as urinary protein excretion of >3.0 g/day and persisting for at least 6 months. Tissue was available for study from both the native kidneys and from the allografts in 36 patients who received 38 grafts. Two patients developed nephrotic syndrome in two consecutive transplants. Both received first kidneys from related donors and second kidneys from cadaveric donors. The follow-up period for functioning allografts ranged from 10 months to 15 years, with a mean follow-up period of 38 ± 5.5 months.

The histopathological criteria we used to determine the type of lesion present in the allografts have been described in detail elsewhere.[7] Twenty-eight of the 36 patients had glomerular diseases as the cause of renal failure in their native kidneys, and eight had diseases that did not primarily affect the glomeruli such as polycystic kidney disease, obstructive uropathy, medullary cystic disease, and tubulointerstitial nephritis. Seven of the 28 patients with glomerular disease had focal segmental glomerulosclerosis (FSG), five had type I membranoproliferative GN (MPGN), five had membranous nephropathy, five had proliferative GN and six had unclassifiable glomerular diseases with either atypical glomerular abnormalities or far advanced sclerotic glomerular changes. The three major groups of abnormalities identified in the transplanted kidneys in these patients were allograft glomerulopathy, recurrent GN, and *de novo* GN.

The seven patients with FSG received nine allografts, and FSG recurred in four of the grafts. All five patients with type I MPGN developed this lesion in their allograft, and three of them had, in addition, changes consistent with allograft glomerulopathy. All of the allografts in patients with membranous nephropathy had allograft nephropathy, and none developed recurrent disease. Three allografts in patients with proliferative glomerulonephritis revealed allograft nephropathy, and two developed membranous nephropathy with subepithelial deposits. Of the six allografts in patients who had glomerular disease that could not be classfied, four had allograft nephropathy, one had membranous nephropathy, and one had a minimal-change lesion.

All of the eight patients with nonglomerular disease had only allograft nephropathy identified. Thus, the alterations in 38 renal allografts with the nephrotic syndrome were allograft glomerulopathy in 25 (65.8%), recurrent GN in nine (23.7%), and *de novo* GN in four (10.5%).

Of interest was the observation that graft survival in patients who developed nephrotic syndrome differed markedly depending on the type of lesion found. The patients with recurrent disease, either FSG or MPGN, had a rapidly progressive course with loss of renal function within 1–2 years. There was no relationship between the tempo of progression of the original kidney disease and the recurrent disease, which tended to be much more rapid. Immunologically mediated experimental renal disease progresses more rapidly in animals with decreased renal mass,[8] and our findings suggest that a similar phenomenon may occur in man. The patients who developed *de novo* GN became nephrotic 2–3 years after transplantation; these grafts functioned for at least 3 years, and one continues to function at 15 years. This patient has, in fact, had three normal pregnancies during this time. The patients who developed allograft nephropathy alone had a course somewhere between these two extreme, half of them losing their grafts by about 3 years.

FOCAL SEGMENTAL GLOMERULOSCLEROSIS IN TRANSPLANTED KIDNEYS

Although primary FSG is a lesion that may recur following transplantation, it is an alteration that is also found with a variety of other diseases, including hypertension,[9] poststreptococcal GN,[10] focal proliferative GN,[11] reflux nephropathy,[12-14] heroin-associated nephropathy,[15] and idiopathic nephrotic syndrome.[16-18] Focal segmental glomerulosclerosis may also be found in allografts of patients whose original disease was other than FSG.[19,20] We therefore examined biopsy material from 154 transplants (138 patients) taken 3 weeks to 48 months after transplant in patients with progressive azotemia, nephrotic syndrome, or hematuria to investigate the incidence, clinicopathological significance, and pathogenesis of FSG in renal transplant recipients.[21]

The essential histological criteria for the diagnosis of FSG were focal (less than 50% of the glomeruli) and segmental solidification, collapse, sclerosis, and/or hyalinosis of the glomerular tufts. The diagnosis of FSG was made when the changes in the biopsies met these criteria, even if other abnormalities were present. The nonspecific glomerular changes found in kidneys with FSG were variable and included an increased mesangial matirix, mesangial cell proliferation, shrinkage of glomerular tufts, irregular thickening, wrinkling, or splitting of the basement membrane, and epithelial foot process effacement.

Among the 154 allografts studies, FSG was identified in 18. This lesion was found as early as 3 weeks and as late as 43 months after transplant, but it was more common in grafts that had survived for at least 6 months. Thirteen of the 138 patients who received these 154 grafts had FSG as their primary renal disease, and received 16 grafts. Four of these patients developed FSG in their transplants (30.8%), and two developed it in two consecutive transplants. These patients were also nephrotic and were included in the study mentioned above. The remaining 125 patients who did not have FSG as their original kidney disease received 138 kidney transplants, and FSG was found in 12 of the kidneys. The distribution of affected glomeruli was quite different in patients who presumably had recurrent FSG than in those who developed *de novo* FSG. In the former group, the lesions were predominantly in the juxtamedullary glomeruli, whereas in the latter the lesions were located predominantly in the outer cortical glomeruli. The patients with *de novo* FSG also had more severe vascular lesions and more extensive interstitial fibrosis. Immunofluorescent studies revealed focal granular deposits of immunoglobulins (IgG and IgM), C3, and fibrin in the mesangium and various other locations in the glomeruli and did not distinguish between the two groups.

The clinical features of the two groups also differed. Patients with recurrent FSG had a higher incidence of hypertension, hematuria, nephrotic sydrome, and azotemia than did those patients with *de novo* FSG.

Our findings support the hypothesis that alterations in the intrarenal vasculature related to chronic rejection may be a major factor in the pathogenesis and progression of *de novo* FSG in renal allografts. These vascular changes primarily take the form of an obliterative arteriolitis, resulting in glomerular ischemia. Direct injury to segments of glomerular tufts may also occur secondary to cellular or humoral allograft reactions.

Focal segmental glomerulosclerosis is seen in kidneys of some patients with vesicoureteral reflux.[12-14] Among the patients whom we studied, five had reflux into the transplanted kidney, but none of these developed FSG.

PROTEINURIA AND HYPERTENSION IN PATIENTS WITH LONG-STANDING TRANSPLANTS

Patients with kidney transplants have a total renal mass that is less than normal, and their kidneys are subject to recurrent immunologic injury. In addition to the other problems associated with transplantation, these kidneys may also be subject to renal injury related to hyperperfusion. It was of interest, therefore, to determine the incidence of proteinuria, hypertension, and azotemia in patients who had renal grafts that had been functioning for several years and had minimal evidence of immunologic injury.

Fifty-one patients with functioning grafts followed in our clinic for more than 5 years were studied. Thirteen of the grafts were from related living donors, and 38 were from cadaveric donors. The average age of the patients at the time of transplant was 33.5 ± 12. Immediately after transplant, only 12 patients were normotensive, whereas at the end of 5 years, 20 (39%) were normotensive, requiring no antihypertensive agents. Only one patient was normotensive in the first posttransplant year and subsequently became hypertensive 2.5 years post-transplant. Among the patients who were hypertensive at 5 years (31 patients), 20 were easily controlled with antihypertensive therapy. The incidence of proteinuria did not change appreciably during the first 5 years posttransplant. Sixty-one percent of the patients had insignificant proteinuria in the first posttransplant year, and 55% in the fifth year. One patient had >3 g of urinary protein per 24 h in the first transplant year, and an additional three patients developed nephrotic-range proteinuria by 5 years. The remaining 47 patients had less than 900 mg urinary protein per 24 h. Most patients with significant proteinuria (>3 g per 24 h) lose their kidneys within the first 5 years with rejection, recurrent disease, or *de novo* glomerulonephritis. Of those who maintain kidney function, there is not yet a discernable trend towards increasing hypertension or proteinuria.

PROTEINURIA, HYPERTENSION, AND AZOTEMIA IN KIDNEY DONORS

Two hundred sixty-one living related donor transplants have been done at The New York Hospital–Cornell Medical Center between 1963 and 1982. Recently, two of the donors have come to our attention because of the development of nephrotic syndrome and azotemia. One patient is a 36–year–old male who had donated a kidney to his brother 13 years ago and noted edema approximately 12 years later. He was hypertensive and azotemic with a urinary protein excretion of 21 g per 24 h. Renal biopsy revealed two-thirds of the glomeruli to be sclerotic, and the remainder showed a spectrum of changes including a diffuse expansion of the mesangium, areas of focal and generalized proliferation, and membranoproliferative changes in some glomeruli. Acute and chronic interstitial disease was also present. Scattered deposits of IgG, and C3 were found on immunofluorescent staining. This patient also had a history of intravenous drug abuse, and the pathological changes were consistent with heroin-associated nephropathy. The second patient is a 63-year-old female who donated a kidney to her son 13 years ago and has had pedal edema for the past year. She was found to be nephrotic with a urinary protein excretion of 11 g per 24 h and a creatinine clearance about 50% of normal. This patient refused a renal biopsy and was treated with steroids with a decrease in urinary protein and an improvement in renal function.

Although these kidney diseases could be unrelated to uninephrectomy, we systematically evaluated renal function in as many donors as could be located. So far, approximately 40 people who donated kidneys 2–15 years ago have been studied. The results of this study will soon be reported. The tentative conclusions that can be drawn from the preliminary data are that about one-third of uninephrectomized patients have mild hypertension, not significantly different from a control group. Minimal proteinuria is seen, as is a slight increase in serum creatinine. Whether or not the significant renal disease we found in two donors is related to nephrectomy, or whether idiopathic disease was accentuated by the loss of renal mass is not known. Clearly, data on donors must be expanded so that informed decisions can be made on the risks of kidney donation. This is an especially acute problem now, since in our program, using donor-specific transfusions, the graft success rate is >95%.

ACKNOWLEDGMENT. Many physicians actively participated in the long-term evaluation of these patients and provided constant advice and guidance about their management and the evaluation of proteinuria. We especially acknowledge the contributions of Drs. Albert L. Rubin, Robert R. Riggio, Manikkam Suthanthiran, Luis Tapia, John Sullivan, Stuart Saal, Jacqueline Chami, and William T. Stubenbord.

REFERENCES

1. Brenner BM, Meyer TW, Hostetter TW: Dietary protein intake and the progressive nature of kidney disease: The role of hemodynamically mediated glomerular injury in the pathogenesis of progressive glomerular sclerosis in aging, renal ablation, and intrinsic renal disease. *N Engl J Med* 307:652–659, 1982
2. Cheigh JS, Stenzel KH, Rubin AL: Low dose immunosuppressive therapy in kidney transplantation. *Transplant* 34:232–233, 1982
3. Suthanthiran M, Garovoy MR: Immunologic monitoring of the renal transplant recipient. *Urol Clin North Am* 10:315–325, 1983
4. Masur H, Cheigh JS, Stubenbord WT: Infection following renal transplantation: A changing pattern. *Rev Infect Dis* 4:1208–1219, 1982
5. Revillard JP, Manuel Y, Betuel H, et al: Proteinuria in human renal allografts—sequential studies, in Manuel Y, Revillard JP, Betuel H (eds): *Proteins in Normal and Pathological Urine*. Baltimore, University Park Press, 1970, p 309
6. Laterre EC, Van Ypersele De Strihou C, Alexandre GPJ: Proteinuria in human renal allograft with special reference to glomerular permeability in acute rejection crisis, in Manuel Y, Revillard JP, Betuel H (eds): *Proteins in Normal and Pathological Urine*. Baltimore, University Park Press, 1970, p 300
7. Cheigh JS, Mouradian J, Susin M, et al: Kidney transplant nephrotic syndrome: Relationship between allograft histopathology and natural course. *Kidney Int* 18:358–365, 1983
8. Beyer MM, Steinberg AD, Nicastri AD, et al: Unilateral nephrectomy: Effect on survival in NZB/NZB mice. *Science* 198:511–513, 1977
9. Sommers SC, Relman AS, Smithwich RH: Histologic studies of kidney biopsy specimens from patients with hypertension. *Am J Pathol* 34:685–715, 1958
10. Gallo GR, Feiner HD, Steele JM jr, et al: Role of intrarenal vascular sclerosis in progression of poststreptococcal glomerulonephritis. *Clin Nephrol* 13:49–57, 1980
11. Whitworth JA, Turner DR, Leibowitz S, et al: Focal segmental sclerosis or scarred focal proliferative glomerulonephritis? *Clin Nephrol* 9:229–234, 1978
12. Kincaid-Smith P: Glomerular and vascular lesions in chronic atrophic pyelonephritis and reflux nephropathy. *Adv Nephrol* 5:3–17, 1975
13. Aladjem M, Schoeneman MJ, Bennet B, et al: Focal segmental glomerulosclerosis with proteinuria and chronic interstitial nephritis. *NY State J Med* 78:579–581, 1978
14. Bhathena DB, Weiss JH, Holland NH, et al: Focal and segmental glomerular sclerosis in reflux nephropathy. *Am J Med* 68:886–892, 1980
15. Sreepada Rao TK, Nicastri AD, Friedman EA: Renal consequences of narcotic abuse. *Adv Nephrol* 7:261–290, 1978
16. Rich AR: A hitherto undescribed vulnerability of the juxtamedullary glomeruli in lipoid nephrosis. *Bull Johns Hopkins Hosp* 100:173–186, 1957

17. Hyman LR, Burkholder PM: Focal sclerosing gomerulonephropathy with segmental hyalinosis. A clinicopathologic analysis. *J Lab Invest* 28:533–544, 1973
18. Habib R: Focal glomerular sclerosis. *Kidney Int* 4:355–361, 1973
19. Mathew TH, Mathews DC, Kincaid-Smith P: Glomerular lesions after renal transplantation. *Am J Med* 59:177–190, 1975
20. Melekzadeh MH, Heuser ET, Ettenger RB, et al: Focal glomerulosclerosis and renal transplantation. *J Pediatr* 95:249–254, 1979
21. Cheigh JS, Mouradian J, Soliman M, et al: Focal segmental glomerulosclerosis in renal transplants. *Am J Kidney Dis* 2:449–454, 1983

10

Proteinuria as Seen by the Urologist

CIRIL J. GODEC

INTRODUCTION

The urologist often sees patients with proteinuria. Although these patients usually seek the advice of a nephrologist, some of them will have urological disease and require a urological diagnostic work-up. Proteinuria is a symptom and almost never a disease in itself. In most cases, proteinuria is a harbinger of a benign renal pathological process. However, in some cases, it can represent the very first clinical symptom of urological malignancy. Therefore, the urologist must evaluate the patient to determine if there is urological pathology causing the proteinuria.

From the urological viewpoint, proteinuria can be divided into two broad categories: those associated with benign conditions and those associated with malignant diseases. Any substantial increase in renal vein pressure can be associated with benign causes of proteinuria. Varicocele can be associated with increased renal vein pressure. In a group of patients with subclinical varicocele, some individuals can have increased levels of protein in the urine, which can be the only symptom of varicocele. Gradual occlusion of the main renal artery does allow the buildup of extensive collateral circulation, which, in turn, may produce proximal ureteral notching. This can be seen distinctly on IVP as a result of dialated ureteral veins. In his elegant study, Wegner et al.[1] described the radiography of renal venous drainages. One drainage system, which applies to both kidneys, is radiographically seen as a subcapsular plexus that connects capsular veins with perirenal veins. The second system is present only on the left side and consists of left adrenal and gonadal veins, which can drain the left renal vein in cases in which the obstruction is close to the vena cava. On this side the left gona-

---

CIRIL J. GODEC • Department of Urology, The Long Island College Hospital, Brooklyn, New York 11201

dal and left adrenal veins drain into the left renal vein; on the right side these veins drain directly into the vena cava.

The precise nature of proteinuria under these circumstances has not yet been documented. Very likely one can link the proteinuria with the presence of intrarenal hypertension. Nevertheless, on animal models Harris et al.[2] found that 6 weeks after the occlusion of the renal vein in dogs, the opposite kidney displayed changes resembling glomerulonephritis as well. All dogs had proteinuria. From this experiment one can conclude that unilateral renal vein thrombosis can produce bilateral membraneous glomerulonephritis. Similar transient proteinuria with nephrotic syndrome was also seen in constrictive pericarditis, tricuspid valve insufficiency, and congestive heart failure. As soon as successful treatment decreases renal vein pressure, the nephrotic syndrome with proteinuria disappears. Renal artery stenosis has been considered a causative factor of idiopathic nephrotic syndrome.[3] Animal models have shown that renin and angiotensin can induce proteinuria.[4] In one recent report of three patients, the proteinuria has been described as being associated with renal arterial occlusion and hyperreninuria. Surgical bypass for arterial stenosis or nephrectomy resulted in a rapid decrease of proteinuria.[5]

INFECTIONS

In some specific urinary tract infections, the degree of proteinuria is correlated with the intensity of infection. This is especially true for endemic infection with Schistosoma haematobium.[6] The precise mechanism of proteinuria in schistosomiasis is not completely clear. It could be secondary to nephritis. In some endemic areas, this infection has been described as being associated with the nephrotic syndrome.

TRAUMA

Another major subset of renal pathology that can present with proteinuria is renal trauma. Although we do not have documentation that renal trauma can directly cause glomerulonephritis, one can speculate that the association between renal trauma and concomitant glomerulonephritis is more than coincidental. Only recently, a case with renal trauma was described in which renal trauma triggered albuminuria and the nephrotic syndrome.[7] Two weeks after trauma, the patient developed massive proteinuria. Radiological examination documented a partially recanalized thrombus in the renal vein of the injured kidney. Renal biopsy was performed on both sides, and acute glomerulonephritis was documented not only on the injured side but also on the contralateral side. Very likely, increased renal venous pressure produced by renal vein thrombosis caused proteinuria and the subsequent nephrotic syndrome. There could be another explanation for proteinuria in renal vein thrombosis: the diminished blood flow could produce microthrombotic changes and deposition of fibrin and its degradation products with circulating immunocomplexes in the glomeruli.[8] These degradation products are chemotactic and could cause accumulation and activation of granulocytes in glomeruli and thus damage the basement membrane.

Although we do not have documentation in the literature that renal trauma can directly trigger glomerulonephritis, we can use some indirect evidence in an attempt to explain the association between renal trauma and glomerulonephritis. Normal glomeruli possess only a trace of albumin (radius 37 Å), which represents only 0.02% of the glomerular filtration rate, e.g., 2 g/day in the adult male. With smaller proteins, the filtration rate increases rapidly and for myoglobin is 37% of GFR. Thus, we can explain why there is almost no protein found in human plasma that is smaller than albumin. Normal glomeruli pass approximately 2–4 g of protein a day, and approximately 50% of these are proteins smaller than albumin.

MALIGNANCY

One of the major areas where the urologist might be dealing with proteinuria is in the presence of urological and nonurological malignancies. Some authors even suggest that every sudden appearance of nephrotic syndrome in an older patient should be followed by an aggressive diagnostic evaluation for potential malignant neoplasm.[9] The invasion of the renal vein by a malignant thrombus in patients with malignant renal cell tumors can be suspected from the presence of proteinuria. In a group of 17 patients, Baum and associates[10] documented the association between the malignant spread into the renal vein or into the vena cava and proteinuria. The 13 patients without renal vein or caval invasion did not have any proteinuria, but four patients with invasion of the renal vein did display significant proteinuria. We recently had three patients with significant proteinuria (3 +), and in two of them proteinuria disappeared after nephrectomy. All three had renal vein involvement (unpublished data). Analysis of proteins obtained from the urine of patients with renal cell tumors documented a protein of 12,000 molecular weight. The same protein was absent from urine obtained from patients without renal cell carcinoma. From its intense red color and specific absorption spectrum, this protein has been identified as a species of cytochrome c. This protein could possibly serve as a useful marker for the early detection of renal cell cancer.

Increased amounts of protein in the urine have been documented in patients with malignancies of the kidneys or urinary pathways.[11,12] It was suggested that proteins, especially immunoglobulins, could be shed from the tumor surface.[13] It was also suggested that patients with bladder cancer produce immune response to malignant bladder cells.[14,15] Antigen–antibody complexes deposited in renal glomeruli have been documented in connection with urothelial malignancies.[16] This glomerular lesion can cause increased protein excretion or even nephrotic syndrome. Proteinuria did correlate well with the grade of transitional cell tumor.[17] In some cases, proteinuria did persist even when patients were tumor free. After radiation treatment for bladder tumors, some patients do develop proteinuria. Although it is not clear what the mechanism is, it is possible that the bladder becomes more permeable for some low-molecular-weight proteins. Similar changes in urothelium might be produced by intravesical chemotherapy.[17]

The nephrotic syndrome was also documented in patients with extrarenal epithelial carcinoma[18] and in patients with malignant lymphoma without renal involvement.[19-21] In general, proteinuria is not an unusual finding in patients with extrarenal malignancies: it might be produced by amyloidosis, direct invasion of renal parenchyma by lymphoma, malignant renal vein thrombus, nephrocalcinosis or compression of the collecting system by retroperitoneal tumors. Tubular obstruction secondary to deposit of uric acid crystals during rapid cellular breakdown during treatment of malignant disease can also be the cause of proteinuria. The renal complications secondary to myelomatosis are well known. Cantrell[22] described a 60-year-old man with nephrotic syndrome that preceded the diagnosis of gastric carcinoma. After gastrectomy, the nephrotic syndrome disappeared completely.

Nephrotic syndrome was also described in patients with bronchial neoplasms[23]; this association could possibly be explained by the close association of lung and kidney in Goodpasture syndrome, where cross-reacting antibodies between lung and basement membrane have been documented. A patient with thyroid carcinoma and renal disease, membranous and glomerular lesion, and proteinuria was described in the Massachusetts General Hospital case records.[24] Another patient with colonic carcinoma was reported to have massive proteinuria, which completely disappeared after successful resection.[23] Renal biopsy in this patient showed documented membranous glomerulopathy.

All the above reports on the association between proteinuria and malignant tumors should make both the urologist and the nephrologist aware that glomerulonephritis of unknown cause or sudden onset of proteinuria might be a very first harbinger of malignant disease, which must be carefully looked at. In 1966, Lee and associates reviewed 101 cases of idiopathic nephroses and found an incidence of cancer in 10.9%, which is far above the expected incidence for the age-matched group in the general population.[18]

The complete description of proteinuria in patients with malignant disease is not yet available. Nevertheless, the clinical evidence based on the limited data at the present time regarding "nonmedical proteinuria" does provide enough warning that proteinuria is found in certain benign or malignant urological conditions to warrant further investigation. Also, the medically unexplained sudden appearance of proteinuria in elderly patients needs additional diagnostic evaluation.

This leads us to the conclusion that proteinuria is an early messenger for a multitude of urological disorders, including neoplastic disease, and that the role of the urologist in this setting will increase with time.

REFERENCES

1. Wegner GP, Crummy AB, Flaherty TT, et al: Renal vein thrombosis: A roentgenographic diagnosis. *Jama* 209:1661 1969
2. Harris JD, Ehrenfeld, Wylie E: Experimental renal vein thrombosis. *Surg Gynecol Obstet* 126:555 1968
3. Shapiro AP, McDonald RH, Sheib E: Renal artery stenosis and hypertension. *Am J Cardiol* 37:1035 1976
4. Addis T, Barret E, Boyd RJ, et al: Renin proteinuria in the rat: 1) The relation between the proteinuria and the pressor effect of renin. *J Exp Med* 89:131 1949
5. Kumar A, Shapiro AP: Proteinuria and nephrotic syndrome induced by renin in patients with renal artery stenosis. *Arch Intern Med* 140:1631 1980
6. Mott KE, Dixon H: Relation between the intensity of *Schistosoma haematobium* infection and clinical hematuria and proteinuria. *Lancet* 1:1005 1983
7. Laauso M, Pentiuainen PJ, Lampainen E, et al: Trauma, renal vein thrombosis and subsequent nephrotic syndrome. *Ann Clin Res* 14:140 1982
8. Brenner BN, Rector FC, (eds): *The Kidney* Philadelphia, WB Saunders, 1976, p 894
9. Loughridge LW, Lewis MG: Nephrotic syndrome in malignant disease of non-renal origin. *Lancet* 1:256 1971
10. Baum NH, Mobley DF, Carlton CE Jr.: Renal vein thrombosis in renal cell carcinoma. Proteinuria as a diagnostic sign. *Urology* 16:131 1982
11. Harvey NA: A clinical and pathological study with special reference to the "hypernephrotic" tumors. *J Urol* 57:669 1947
12. Hemmigsen L, Skaarup P: Urinary excretion of ten plasma proteins in patients with extrarenal epithelial carcinoma. *Acta Chir Scand* 143:177 1977
13. Johansson B, Kistner S: Proteinuria in patients with uroepithelial tumors with special

regards to tumor size, clinical staging and grade of malignancy. *Scand J Urol Nephrol* 9:45 1975

14. Catalona WJ: Commentary on the immuno-biology of bladder cancer. *J Urol* 118:2 1977
15. Jones LW, Levin A, Fudenberg HH: Glomeral antigen complexes associated with transitional cell carcinoma. *Surg Gynecol Obstet* 140:896 1975
16. Hemmingsen L, Rasmussen F, Skaarup P, et al: Urinary protein profiles in patients with urothelial bladder tumors. *Br J Urol* 53:324 1981
17. Yu H, Glasman MRG, Robinson B, et al: Changes in the urine protein profile following intravesical doxorubicin. *J Urol* 128:272 1982
18. Lee JC, Yamauchi H, Hopper J: The association of cancer and nephrotic syndrome. *Ann Intern Med* 64:41 1966
19. Ghosh L, Muehrcue RC: The nephrotic syndrome: A prodrome to lymphoma. *Ann Intern Med* 72:379 1970
20. Hyman LR, Burckholder PM, Joo PA, et al: Malignant lymphoma and nephrotic syndrome. *J Pediatr* 82:207 1973
21. Sherman RL, Susin M, Weusler ME, et al: Lipoid nephrosis in Hodgkin's disease. *Am J Med* 52:699 1972
22. Cantrell EG: Nephrotic syndrome caused by removal of gastric carcinoma. *Br J Med* 2:739 1969
23. Hopper J. Jr.: Tumor related renal lesions. *Ann Intern Med* 81:550 1974
24. Castleman B: Case records of the Massachusetts General Hospital. Case 29-1963. *N Engl J Med* 268:943 1963

Part III

Pathophysiological Consequences and Management of Proteinuria

In this section, Schreiner and Glassock, two pioneer researchers in proteinuria, broach key questions vital to the full understanding of the pathophysiological and clinical consequences of urinary protein loss. These two essays proffer both basic and clinical insights to the issue, "What is proteinuria?" Schreiner's work clarifies differences in glomerular pathology in proteinuric states in which >3.5 g are excreted daily compared with a daily excretion of <2 g. Validation of Schreiner's thesis that proteinuria occurs in a bimodal distribution—large (>3/5 g) and small (<2.0 g) daily amounts according to diagnosis—ought to be a near-term clinical goal now that we can employ semiquantitative measurements of proteinuria using reagent strips with color changes proportional to the amount of protein in solution. It follows that mass screening for proteinuria is now possible. Every student of kidney disease is curious about the genesis of proteinuria and the clues it offers to anatomic diagnosis, prognosis, and specific treatment. As beautifully detailed by Glassock, we know that proteinuria is the final common pathway of many extrarenal and kidney diseases. Glassock assesses the pathophysiological impact of proteinuria on lipid, trace metal, and hormone metabolism. He also makes sense of the confusing coagulation and immunologic abnormalities that accompany heavy proteinuria. Glassock's masterful compilation of the immunologic pertubations of the nephrotic syndrome leave us wanting to know more than he can tell. "It is presently uncertain," Glassock remarks, "whether these abnormalities are merely a consequence of the nephrotic syndrome *per se* or a manifestation of an underlying disturbance in cell-mediated immunity pathogenetically involved in the underlying lesion...."

M.M.A.

Part III

Pathophysiological Consequences and Management of Proteinuria

11

The Pathophysiological Consequences of Heavy Proteinuria

RICHARD J. GLASSOCK

INTRODUCTION

It should be evident that heavy and prolonged urinary protein loss consequent to defects in the permeability of the glomerular capillary wall leads to disturbances well beyond the obvious edema formation. These more covert disturbances may, in many respects, be more clinically important than the largely cosmetic problems of edema. The loss of plasma proteins through a damaged glomerular filter evokes a complex series of circumstances involving lipids, transport proteins, components of coagulation, and immunologic pathways. Each of these, in turn, is associated with clinical features that are as much a part of the nephrotic syndrome as edema and hypoalbuminemia. The purpose of this chapter is to highlight these features in order to emphasize the systemic metabolic, endocrine, and immunologic aspects of the heavy proteinuric state.

THE FUNDAMENTAL ABNORMALITY

The basis of the disturbances accompanying the nephrotic syndrome is, of course, the excessive movement of circulating plasma proteins into Bowman's space. According to current concepts of glomerular permselectivity (described by B. M. Brenner and L. D. Dworkin, chapter 1, this volume), the plasma protein species that will escape into Bowman's space will depend, at least, on the relative degree of abnormality of the charge-selective and size-selective barriers of the glomerular capillary wall.[1]

RICHARD J. GLASSOCK • Department of Medicine, UCLA School of Medicine, Harbor-UCLA Medical Center, Torrance, California 90509.

Accordingly, a selective disturbance of the anionic constituents of the glomerular capillary wall (e.g., minimal-change disease)[2] would be expected to be associated with disproportionate losses of anionic plasma proteins of intermediate molecular weight (e.g., albumin), whereas structural damage to the integrity of the glomerular capillary wall associated with defects of the size-selective barrier would be associated with the loss of more neutral and higher-molecular-weight proteins in addition to albumin. These differing patterns may be associated with various metabolic and endocrine disturbances. Once filtered through the defective glomerular capillary wall, these plasma proteins will be reabsorbed and catabolized in the proximal tubule to a varying degree (see C.H. Park *et al.*, chapter 3, this volume). Thus, the measurement of urinary losses of individual proteins may not truly reflect their rate of egress from the circulation and into Bowman's space. However, since in states of massive proteinuria the glomerular losses greatly exceed the tubular reabsorptive maxima, the fractional excretion of filtered proteins is ordinarily quite high. If tubular reabsorption is nonselective, then the large load of filtered albumin may also effectively compete for reabsorption with other proteins normally present in small quantities in the tubular fluid, thus depressing their reabsorption rates.

The loss of plasma proteins would be accompanied by a reduction in plasma concentration and in the intravascular and/or extravascular pool sizes in every case were it not for the body's capacity to augment cellular synthesis in response to perceived deficits. The response to urinary albumin loss is the best studied, and because of the central role of hypoalbuminemia in many of the clinical manifestations of nephrotic syndrome, a brief recapitulation of the metabolic response to excessive urinary loss of albumin is in order.

First, as indicated above, the loss of albumin from intravascular and extravascular pools is the result of both excessive urinary excretion and enhanced renal catabolism. In fact, in some situations, the enhanced renal catabolism of filtered albumin may be quantitatively more important than urinary losses.[3] Losses of albumin at other sites, principally the gastrointestinal tract,[4] may occur in severely edematous states. Thus, the fractional catabolic rate of albumin is almost invariably increased in nephrotic syndrome.[3, 5-7] However, because of hypoalbuminemia and reduced albumin pool size, the absolute albumin catabolic rate is either normal or reduced.[8]

Second, hepatic albumin synthesis is increased, although the magnitude of the increase is usually small relative to the degree of hypoalbuminemia.[6, 9, 10] The degree of the increase may be dependent on adequacy of protein intake and on the provision of essential amino acids and calories.[9, 10] The relative roles of enhanced fractional catabolism, amino acid deficiency, and glucocorticoids in the inappropriately low hepatic synthetic response are unclear. However, it is likely that an altered synthetic rate of plasma protein may contribute to the diminution of plasma concentration.

Third, the disturbances in Starling forces in the peripheral capillary consequent to reduction of plasma oncotic pressure lead to accumulation of excessive quantities of interstitial fluid containing a measureable amount of albumin,[8] albeit less than the plasma concentration. Thus, the extravascular pool of albumin enlarges at the expense of the intravascular pool. Some diseases associated with heavy proteinuria may have an additional complicating defect in systemic capillary permeability, further altering the intravascular/extravascular pool size ratios.

LIPID DISORDERS

That excessive fat content of blood frequently but not invariably accompanies heavy proteinuria has been recognized for over three-quarters of a century.[10] The precise nature of the changes in blood lipids accompanying nephrotic syndrome has been extensively studied, and we now have a more or less comprehensive understanding of the mechanisms that underlie these alterations.[8]

First, the increased hepatic synthesis of albumin occurring consequent to enhanced urinary loss and/or renal catabolism leads to an increase in hepatic lipoprotein synthesis *pari passu*.[11,12] The proximal stimulus to hepatic lipoprotein synthesis is in all likelihood not the plasma albumin concentration *per se* but may well be the plasma oncotic pressure or the hepatic interstitial oncotic pressure.[8, 13] in any case, the very-low-density lipoprotein (VLDL) synthesis rate parallels that of albumin synthesis.

Second, although triglyceride-rich VLDL are normally converted to intermediate-density lipoprotein (IDL) and nascent high-density lipoproteins (HDL) in extrahepatic tissue by the action of lipoprotein lipase (LPL),[8] there is evidence that this conversion rate is slowed in nephrotic syndrome, perhaps related to a deficiency in LPL.[14] Furthermore, activation of LPL is dependent on the apolipoprotein C-II content of VLDL.[15] This apolipoprotein is transferred via HDL formed by the action of lecithin–cholesterol acyltransferase (LCAT) on nascent HDL.[8,16] Evidence exists that LCAT deficiency, either from urinary losses or the failure of albumin to remove lysolecithin, an inhibitor of LCAT, may also occur in nephrotic syndrom.[17,18] Urinary losses of glycosoaminoglycans (orosomucoid), which are naturally occurring stimulators of LPL, may also be involved in the depressed activity of LPL in nephrotic syndrome.[19] The failure of LCAT to provide sufficient apolipoprotein C-II to VLDL may deprive the already reduced level of LPL of its naturally occurring activator. In addition, with hypoalbuminemia, free fatty acids (FFA) may accumulate intracellularly and inhibit LPL directly. Correction of hypoalbuminemia with infusion of hyperoncotic albumin may directly enhance the action of LPL.[20] Finally, the formation of HDL by LCAT also subserves an important function of assisting in the removal of cholesterol from the circulation via the bile.

Third, the IDL are normally converted to cholesterol-rich triglyceride-poor low-density lipoproteins (LDL) in the liver and circulation. These LDL are taken up by the liver and peripheral tissues by specific LDL receptors, and the cholesterol is used for intracellular synthesis of cholesterol-dependent membrane material. The LDL receptors are subject to feedback inhibition depending on the level of intracellular cholesterol. Thus, if LDL is produced in excess, the density of the LDL receptors may decrease, further impairing removal of LDL from the circulation. Conversion of IDL to LDL is impaired in nephrotic syndrome,[21] a phenomenon that could conceivably be related to a deficiency in LCAT.[22]

Fourth, HDL is formed by the action of LCAT on nascent HDL, and excessive quantities of HDL may be lost in the urine of some patients with heavy proteinuria.[23, 24] This may lead to a lowered plasma HDL level. Since HDL function is to salvage cholesterol from cells and transport it to the liver and, secondarily, to provide apo-C-II for VLDL activation of LPL, HDL deficiency may accelerate the elevation of total plasma cholesterol levels and further impair conversion of VLDL to LDL.[8]

These complex series of events lead to differing patterns of hyperlipidemia and hyperlipoproteinemia in nephrotic syndrome, dependent on the nature of the underlying glomerular disturbance.[21,25-27] In mild nephrotic syndrome of short duration, the principal change is an elevation of total cholesterol with a modest rise in total triglycerides. The principal abnormality is therefore an increase in LDL and, to a lesser extent, HDL.[27] As the severity of hypoalbuminemia worsens, total cholesterol levels continue to rise, and triglyceride concentrations increase appreciably, particularly when serum albumin concentration is <1 g/dl.[21,27] Thus, with severe and prolonged nephrotic syndrome, the principal abnormality is a rise in VLDL and, to a lesser extent, LDL; HDL levels may, in fact, decline.[21,27]

·Total free fatty acid levels are normal, but the unbound fraction rises inversely with the degree of hypoalbuminemia. Levels of VLDL, IDL, LDL, and HDL cholesterol may all be elevated in the nephrotic syndrome at various stages in the evolution of the underlying disease, and among patients with similar levels of total plasma cholesterol, the proportion accounted for by these varying classes of lipoproteins may differ.[27] For example, in mild to moderate nephrotic syndrome, as stated above, the predominant change is a rise in LDL and HDL cholesterol. In more profound nephrotic syndrome, VLDL and IDL cholesterol increase disproportionately to LDL, and HDL cholesterol levels may fall as a result of excessive urinary loss. Thus, the ratio of LDL to HDL cholesterol may vary widely in patients with nephrotic syndrome even despite equivalent levels of total cholesterol. The lipoprotein electrophoretic patterns observed in nephrotic syndrome, which are dependent on their apolipoprotein composition, vary in nephrotic syndrome but are usually type IIA, IIB, or V.[26] These differences must be taken into account in analyzing the clinical significance of altered lipid and lipoprotein metabolism in nephrotic syndrome.

In nephrotic subjects, elevated total plasma cholesterol levels especially when associated with increased LDL/HDL cholesterol ratios, have been shown to constitute a risk factor for premature coronary artery disease.[28,29] However, the impact of the hypercholesterolemic state seen in nephrotic subjects remains the subject of controversy.[30,31] Some authors have failed to note any excess age-corrected mortality from ischemic heart disease in nephrotic syndrome, but others disagree.[30, 31] Clearly, the potential for disease production must be a plasma level–time product and additionally related to the biochemical makeup of the lipoproteins. Subject with increased total cholesterol and increased HDL cholesterol with brief periods of nephrotic syndrome secondary to remissions in exacerbations (e.g., minimal-change disease)[32,33] would presumably be less vulnerable to the adverse effects of hypercholesterolemia than patients with greatly increased total cholesterol and decreased HDL cholesterol and more persisting nephrotic state (e.g., focal and segmental glomerulosclerosis).[8,32]

Management of the hyperlipidemic state in nephrotic syndrome is at best difficult. Correction of the underlying disease is, of course, the best course to follow. Lipid-lowering agents such as clofibrate, cholestyramine, colestipol, and mevinolin are not usually recommended since they may be poorly tolerated or aggravate other metabolic problems. Concomitant hypoalbuminemia increases free clofibrate levels and may be associated with an increased risk of muscle toxicity.[34] Cholestyramine may aggravate an underlying vitamin D deficiency state by producing malabsorption for orally administered vitamin D (see below). Treatment of the increased total cholesterol would not be indicated if HDL cholesterol were also increased. Restriction of dietary cholesterol, although prudent, has little effect on plasma cholesterol level. A high-protein diet could, theoretically, aggravate hepatic VLDL production. Hyperoncotic albumin will transiently lower plasma lipids but is impractical for long-term therapy. Moderate exercise and low doses of alcohol may increase HDL levels. Little information is available concerning the benefit of combined bile acid sequestration in gut with colestipol and inhibition of HMG-CoA reduction with mevinolin in nephrotic syndrome, although such therapy has dramatic hypocholesterolemic effects in familial hypercholesterolemia.

Clearly, much work is needed to identify those patients with nephrotic syndrome who are at greatest risk for the adverse consequences of the hyperlipidemic disorders and to devise safe and effective measures to correct the underlying disturbances independent of reversal of the basic defect in glomerular permeability. Compounds capable of enhancing LPL activity or LCAT activity or inhibiting hepatic VLDL synthesis would be most welcomed.

TRACE METAL DEFICIENCIES

Many metallic substances normally absorbed by the gastrointestinal tract depend on plasma proteins for transport to other organs, where they are utilized in many metabolic pathways. Furthermore, many critical intracellular enzymes are in part metalloproteins, depending on their metal component for optimal activity. Since many of the transport proteins and metalloenzymes are of intermediate molecular weight, it is not surprising that they may be lost in the urine or demonstrate enhanced renal catabolism in states of heavy proteinuria. Only three metals have been scrutinized to any great extent in nephrotic syndrome: copper, zinc, and iron.[35-40]

Plasma copper is almost entirely bound to cerulopasmin (molecular weight 151,000, and urinary ceruloplasmin and urinary copper may be increased in nephrotic syndrome.[35] A lowered plasma copper level is not uncommon in nephrotic states. The clinical consequences of such a copper deficiency are unknown, but it could have untoward effects on collagen cross linking, bone formation, and hair growth.

Zinc metabolism is clearly altered in nephrotic syndrome.[36,40] Plasma zinc levels are consistently reduced, and urinary zinc excretion is variable, either normal or increased. Plasma zinc is bound to albumin or to a zinc-binding globulin. Zinc deficiency may be responsible for some of the abnormalities in cell-mediated immunity described below, although this aspect has been little studied. Dysgeusia, a not uncommon complaint in severely nephrotic patients, may also be related to zinc deficiency. The role of replacement zinc therapy has not been well established in nephrotic syndrome.

Both total iron and iron binding capacity are frequently reduced in nephrotic syndrome. On rare occasions, this may lead to a microcytic, hypochromic anemia resistant to oral and parenteral therapy.[37] Urinary losses of transferrin (molecular weight 80,000) may be very great, and a profound hypotransferrinemia may be responsible for the anemia.[38,39] In addition, small losses of protein-bound iron, on the order of 0.5 mg/day, in the menstruating female may contribute to iron deficiency. Under these circumstances, prophylactic oral iron therapy may be indicated.

TRANSPORT PROTEIN DEFICIENCY
AND HORMONE METABOLISM

Several hormones (thyroxine, cortisol, and cholecalciferol) are bound to plasma proteins (either a specific globulin, albumin, or prealbumin). Urinary loss of these binding proteins may result in disordered hormone metabolism but seldom leads to any obvious clinical symptomatology. These abnormalities are primarily of interest because of the biochemical perturbations that result.

Thyroid hormone disturbances have been well studied by Feinstein and co-workers. Serum levels of thyroxine-binding globulin (TBG), total serum T_4, T_3, and reverse T_3 (rT_3) are all reduced.[41] Furthermore, binding of T_4 and T_3 to TBG may be decreased. These abnormalities lead to a high T_3 uptake ratio, and occasionally to elevated free T_3 and rT_3. Thyroid-stimulating hormone (TSH) and thyroidal radioactive iodine uptake are normal, as is free T_4 by dialysis. The patients are clinically euthyroid. Despite the low total T_3 and T_4 levels, thyroid replacement is thus not indicated.

Cortisol-binding globulin deficiency is not uncommon in severe nephrotic syndrome.[42] The pathophysiological consequences of this alteration are unknown; however, it is possible that the ratio of bound/free cortisol would be decreased, the apparent space of distribution of cortisol increased, and the metabolic clearance rate disturbed. Thus, the plasma levels of free active hormone and/or the tissue response following pharmacological doses of glucocorticoids could be augmented. Since glucocorticoids are used so frequently to treat nephrotic syndrome, this is an area deserving further study.

Finally, since many commonly employed drugs are tightly bound to plasma proteins, chiefly albumin, following absorption from the gastrointestinal tract or parenteral administration, peak levels of the free and metabolically active drugs will often be increased in nephrotic subjects. This could expose such patients to serious side effects related to the free drug concentration. Thus, dosage of many agents highly protein bound must be adjusted to take this effect into account.

One of the most interesting and best-studied hormonal disturbances in nephrotic syndrome is that of cholecalciferol metabolism. Cholecalciferol (CC), produced in the skin or absorbed from the diet, is converted to 25-hydroxycholecalciferol (25-OH CC) in the liver by a specific hydroxylase. The 25-OH CC is the major circulating form of the various hydroxylated products of CC, and it circulates tightly bound to a cholecalciferol-binding protein (molecular weight 65,000). Since this binding globulin is similar in molecular size to albumin, it is not surprising that substantial amounts of 25-OH CC are lost in the urine.[43-47] Plasma levels of total 25-OH CC are reduced consistently in nephrotic syndrome.[43-47] Since the free, unbound portion of circulating 25-OH CC is the natural substrate for the one-hydroxylase enzyme located in the kidney, the synthetic rate of 1,25-OH CC may actually be augmented, although urinary losses may also occur as a result of modest binding of 1,25-OH CC to cholecalciferol-binding globulin.[48]

The balance of somewhat augmented synthesis and continued losses often leads to a modest decline in plasma 1,25-OH CC levels.[48] However, because of reduced plasma binding of 1,25-OH CC, the free, unbound 1,25-OH CC level may be normal.[48] The 24,25-OH CC levels may be reduced in the plasma.[48] The net effect of these abnormalities in cholecalciferol metabolism is to impair gastrointestinal absorption of calcium[43,49] (although not in a consistent manner) and to reduce the responsiveness of the skeleton to parathyroid hormone (PTH), thus leading to a reduced plasma ionized calcium concentration.[50] As a result of the decrease in plasma ionized calcium, a modest degree of secondary hyperparathyroidism will ensue even in the absence of impaired glomerular filtration rate.[43-47] Total plasma calcium levels are reduced not only because of the decrease of plasma albumin concentration but also because of the decrease in plasma ionized calcium.[43-47,50] The degree of decrease in total calcium is somewhat greater than that predicted solely from the reduction in plasma protein concentration. Profound hypocalciuria despite increased levels of PTH is the rule.[51] The effect of these abnormalities on the skeleton is debated, since both normal bone histology and both osteomalacia and osteitis fibrosa cystica have been observed in bone biopsies taken from nephrotic subjects.[46,52]

Nonetheless, since many patients with nephrotic syndrome will eventually evolve into renal failure, the severity and duration of the proteinuria preceding the onset of end-stage renal failure must be taken into account as a potential risk factor in the ultimate development of renal osteodystrophy. At present, the indications for and usage of oral cholecalciferol replacement therapy in nephrotic syndrome have not yet been established. It seems reasonable to augment oral intake of cholecalciferol, the effectiveness of which would be best monitored by plasma ionized calcium and/or PTH levels. Oral 25-OH CC therapy would appear to be the most reasonable preparation.

COAGULATION DISTURBANCES

The tendency for spontaneous thromboembolic episodes among patients with nephrotic syndrome has long been recognized.[53,54] A possible explanation for this phenomenon may be found in the disturbances in the soluble and cellular components of the coagulation–fibrinolysis cascade. Fibrinogen, factor VIII (antihemophilic globulin), total platelet counts, and platelet aggregation *in vitro* are all increased in nephrotic syndrome,[53,55-57] whereas antithrombin III (heparin cofactor), α-anti-one-trypsin, and endothelial prostacyclin-stimulating factor are all reduced.[58,59] The latter deficiencies are presumably caused by urinary losses, whereas the former reflect enhanced synthesis. Deficiency states are more likely to occur with severe proteinuria and significant hypoalbuminemia. Thus, in nephrotic syndrome, the proaggregatory and procoagulant factors are enhanced, whereas antiaggregatory, anticoagulant, and fibrinolytic mechanisms are impaired. When this is superimposed on endothelial injury from immune complexes, hypertension, hyperlipidemia, or venous stasis from edema or inactivity, it is not surprising that nephrotic syndrome is associated with spontaneous thrombosis in either venous or arterial circuits.

With profound urinary losses of factors IX and XI, a procoagulant deficiency may ensue, which may influence the results of *in vitro* tests of the coagulation cascade[60,61] (e.g., partial thromboplastin time, prothrombin time). However, such abnormalities are rarely associated with a bleeding tendency unless uremia is also present.

Although thrombosis in nephrotic syndrome may involve virtually any vessel of the body (e.g., pulmonary artery, radial artery, saphenous vein, renal vein), the most common site is the renal vein.[53,62] The reason for this predilection is unknown, for in general, flow per unit surface area in the renal vein is very high, a factor that should impede thrombosis. Perhaps the unusual predilection of thrombosis in the renal vein is related to the depletion of anticoagulant properties of renal venous blood secondary to glomerular loss of protein or, alternatively, to the return of proaggregatory peptides from tubular reabsorption and catabolism of filtered protein. Whatever the case, renal vein thrombosis appears to be secondary to the nephrotic milieu rather than a primary cause of the nephrotic syndrome itself. Pulmonary embolization may be a serious but rarely lethal complication of renal vein thrombosis or deep venous thrombosis in the thigh or pelvis of a patient with nephrotic syndrome. Spontaneous thrombosis in the pulmonary arterial circulation may also occur, accounting for the occasional case in which pulmonary "embolism" or infarction has been diagnosed from the findings on ventilation or perfusion scanning of the lung and in whom neither renal vein thrombosis nor peripheral deep venous thrombosis can be documented by invasive or noninvasive means. The overall prevalence of pulmonary embolism or pulmonary thombosis in nephrotic syndrome is not known, but, according to personal experience, it is a rather uncommon event.

The prevalence of renal vein thrombosis in nephrotic syndrome is debated extensively.[53] Llach has described a prevalence of renal vein thrombosis of approximately 22% among among 151 carefully studied cases of nephrotic syndrome (Table I).[53,63] The risk of developing renal vein thrombosis was greatly different between idiopathic and secondary forms of nephrotic syndrome. Overall, one of four patients with idiopathic nephrotic syndrome had evidence of renal vein thrombosis, whereas only one of ten patients with secondary forms of nephrotic syndrome could be demonstrated to have renal vein thrombosis. These prevalence figures may, in all likelihood, be overestimates of the true prevalence, since radiographic assessment of renal vein thrombosis is difficult and may be falsely positive. Furthermore, patients with nephrotic syndrome are more frequently studied angiographically only after symptoms of thromboembolism have ensued. Another problem complicating interpretation of point prevalence studies of renal vein thrombosis in nephrotic syndrome is that we do not know the natural history of the renal vein thrombosis itself. Episodes of renal vein thrombosis with spontaneous resolution may be a relatively common event in nephrotic syndrome.

Whatever the true state of affairs is, it is noteworthy that the risk of renal vein thrombosis is not equal among all of the histopathological variants of secondary and idiopathic nephrotic syndrome. Amyloidosis and systemic lupus erythematosus account for 60% of all reported cases of renal vein thrombosis in secondary forms of nephrotic syndrome, whereas membranous glomerulonephritis and membranoproliferative glomerulonephritis account for the vast majority of reported cases of re-

Table I. Renal Vein Thrombosis: Prevalence in Nephrotic Syndrome[a]

All cases	33/151	21.8%
Idiopathic only	29/110	26%
Membranous or membranoproliferative GN	26/70	37.1%
Other	3/40	7.5%
Secondary only	4/41	9.6%

[a]From Llach,[77] with permission.

nal vein thrombosis occurring in idiopathic nephrotic syndrome. The occurrence of renal vein thrombosis in membranous glomerulopathy is about three times that of membranoproliferative glomerulonephritis and six times more common than that observed in focal sclerosis, minimal-change disease, or mesangial proliferative glomerulonephritis. A high prevalence of renal vein thrombosis has also been noted in experimental membranous glomerulopathy.[64] The reported prevalence of renal vein thrombosis among patients with membranous glomerulopathy studied prospectively, i.e., without regard to the symptoms of thromboembolism, has varied widely. The reasons underlying the broad range of reported prevalence rates of renal vein thrombosis in membranous glomerulopathy (5% to 54%) are unknown but could be related to factors such as duration of disease, antecedent glucocorticoid therapy, or subtle differences in interpretation of renal venous angiograms.

It should be pointed out, however, that the incidence of major thromboembolic episodes in a large population of well-studied patients with membranous glomerulopathy followed prospectively was very low (less than one episode per 100 patients per year) (C. H. Coggins, unpublished data). Furthermore, the effect of chronic asymptomatic unilateral or bilateral renal vein thrombosis on the clinical course of renal disease remains uncertain. Although acute, symptomatic renal vein thrombosis does occur in patients with nephrotic syndrome and may be associated with a dramatic increase in proteinuria, abnormal urinary sediment, and declining glomerular filtration rate, this complication is quite uncommon. Acute renal vein thrombosis occurred in fewer than 10% of the cases of renal vein thrombosis reported by Llach.[53] Chronic renal vein thrombosis is nearly always asymptomatic and unassociated with any dramatic differences in proteinuria or renal function when compared to patients with nephrotic syndrome in the absence of renal vein thrombosis.[65] Thus, the only way to "establish" a diagnosis of renal vein thrombosis in a patient with nephrotic syndrome is by the performance of a renal venous angiogram, a procedure that is not without risk of inducing renal failure or thromboembolism in patients with nephrotic syndrome.

High-resolution two-dimensional ultrasound or digital subtraction angiography may also be of some value in the diagnosis of renal vein thrombosis, but the sensitivity and specificity of these procedures in the diagnosis of renal vein thrombosis are still largely unknown.

Long-term anticoagulants are indicated in those patients with nephrotic syndrome who develop thromboembolic episodes regardless of the site of thrombosis. Heparin may be less effective in those patients with severe antithrombin III deficiency. Since the risk of thromboembolism remains for as long as severe hypoalbuminemia is present, a nephrotic patient who has had one episode of thromboembolism should be treated with anticoagulants for as long as the heavy proteinuria is present, unless, of course, hemorrhagic complications of anticoagulation or uremia ensues.

In this regard, it should be remembered that the metabolic fate of anticoagulant drugs may be altered in nephrotic syndrome, and careful adjustment of dosage is mandatory. Substitution of low-dose aspirin plus dipyridamole or sulfinpyrazone might be indicated for those patients who have difficulty with bleeding complications from anticoagulants yet have a history of recurrent thromboembolism. Long-term anticoagulation is also indicated in the therapy of acute symptomatic renal vein thrombosis with or without pulmonary thromboembolism.[65] The role of long-term anticoagulants in the prevention and therapy of chronic asymptomatic renal vein thrombosis in the absence of pulmonary embolism remains an unsettled issue.

Furthermore, it remains controversial whether prophylactic anticoagulants should be administered to nephrotic subjects to prevent pulmonary embolization or thrombosis regardless of their effect on the occurrence of renal vein thrombosis. The value of such a prophylactic approach would depend on the true risk of renal vein thrombosis and/or pulmonary embolism or thrombosis in nephrotic patients, the likelihood of deterioration of renal function resulting directly from renal vein thrombosis, and the risks of serious bleeding from long-term anticoagulants.

On balance, and until appropriately designed prospective studies are conducted, I would currently not recommend prophylactic anticoagulants in all cases of idiopathic nephrotic syndrome or in those with membranous glomerulopathy or membranoproliferative glomerulonephritis. Similarly, unless patients have experienced a clinical thromboembolic event, I cannot justify a "routine" search for covert, chronic renal vein thrombosis in patients with idiopathic nephrotic syndrome including those with membranous glomerulopahty. If, however, a renal venous angiogram is performed in a patient with nephrotic syndrome who has not experienced a clinical thromboembolic event and the study unequivocally demonstrates a unilateral or bilateral renal vein thrombosis, it would seem prudent to treat with anticoagulants for several months. If a repeat study should show recanalization, or if the nephrotic syndrome has abated in the meantime, anticoagulation could be safely discontinued. if the nephrotic syndrome persists and anticoagulants are discontinued, it seems likely that renal vein thrombosis will recur. If simple, accurate, inexpensive, and safe noninvasive methods for the detection of renal vein thrombosis can be developed (e.g., plasma β-thromboglobulin assays, high-resolution ultrasound), then it might be worthwhile to screen all newly diagnosed patients with membranous glomerulopathy and membranoproliferative glomerulonephritis for covert renal vein thrombosis.

IMMUNOLOGIC ABNORMALITIES

The perturbations in humoral and cellular immunity and the mediators of inflammation and tissue repair that occur in nephrotic syndrome are receiving increasing attention. Acquired hypogammaglobulinemia is very common in nephrotic syndrome, perhaps primarily because of increased urinary loss or greatly enhanced renal catabolism.[66, 67] It is also possible that active endogenous suppression of IgG synthesis may account for the acquired IgG deficiency in some forms of nephrotic syndrome.[68] Serum IgG levels are profoundly diminished in minimal-change disease, a condition in which urinary losses of IgG are minimal[69,70] (C. H. Coggins, unpublished data).

Active, monocyte-dependent suppression of IgG synthesis has also been described in membranous glomerulopathy.[68] Interestingly, the depression of IgG levels may preferentially affect only certain subclasses of IgG.[69] A charge-selective defect in the glomerular capillary wall would likely enhance the urinary excretion of the more anionic or neutral IgG classes while retarding the filtration of the more cationic IgG classes.[2] The IgG deficiency may result in increased susceptibility to infection with gram-negative or gram-positive organisms, particularly *Streptococcus pneumoniae*, *E. coli*, *Klebsiella aerobacter*, and *Hemophilus*. The plasma levels of other immunoglobulins (IgM, IgA, IgE) may be increased in certain forms of nephrotic syndrome.[70] For example, IgM and/or IgE levels may be increased in minimal-change disease,[70,71] whereas IgA levels may be increased in patients with Buerger's disease presenting with nephrotic syndrome.[72]

In general, serum levels of complement components are normal in nephrotic syndrome except for membranoproliferative glomerulonephritis, SLE, cryoimmunoglobulinemia, and acute and chronic infections in which C3 and other early acting components of the classical cascade may be decreased by either peripheral consumption or impaired monocyte synthesis or both.[73] A slight reduction in C1q, roughly correlated with the extent of depression of IgG is frequently seen in minimal-change disease.[73] C3 levels are nearly always normal in minimal-change disease, focal glomerulosclerosis, and membranous glomerulopathy.[73] C1r, C1s, C2, and C4 deficiency may be seen in SLE, but this is not an effect of nephrotic syndrome but rather reflects a genetic abnormality in the structural gene responsible for the synthesis of these complement proteins. Factor B, a component of the alternate pathway of complement activation, may be lost in the urine and account for a decline in the plasma level.[74] Such a deficiency of factor B may account for an impaired opsonization of bacteria.

Cell-mediated immunity may be abnormal in nephrotic syndrome, at least when assessed by a variety of *in vitro* assays. Phytohemagglutinin- and antigen-induced blastogenesis and mixed leukocyte culture reactivity are impaired in nephrotic syndrome.[75,76] These findings could reflect the accumulation of immunoregulatory IDL and LDL in the plasma, circulating immune complexes, the occurrence of lymphocytotoxic antibody, the loss of cofactors necessary for optimal growth of cells in culture in the urine, or concomitant zinc deficiency. In some instances, enhanced T-cell-mediated suppression is responsible for the observed abnormality. It is presently uncertain whether these abnormalities are merely a consequence of the nephrotic state *per se* or whether they represent a manifestation of an underlying disturbance in cell-mediated immunity pathogenetically involved in the underlying lesion responsible for nephrotic syndrome. The *in vitro* abnormalities of cell-mediated immunity do not seem to be related to any unusual prevalence of obligate intracellular infections such as tuberculosis or to an increased prevalence of malignancy.

REFERENCES

1. Brenner BM, Hostetter TH, Humes HD: Molecular basis of proteinuria of glomerular origin. *N Engl J Med* 298:826–833, 1979
2. Carrie BJ, Salyer WR, Myers BD: Minimal change nephropathy: An electrochemical disorder of the glomerular basement membrane. *Am J Med* 70:262–271, 1981
3. Kaitz AL: Albumin metabolism in nephrotic adults. *J Lab Clin Med* 53:186, 1959
4. Jensen H, Jarnum S, Hart Jansen JP: Gastrointestinal protein loss and intestinal function in the nephrotic syndrome. *Nephron* 3:209, 1966

5. Gitlin D, Janeway CA, Farr LE: Studies on the metabolism of plasma proteins in the nephrotic syndrome. I. Albumin, γ-globulin and iron-binding globulin. *J Clin Invest* 35:44, 1956

6. Jensen H: Plasma protein and lipid pattern in the nephrotic syndrome. *Acta Med Scand* 182:465, 1967

7. Johansson SV, Odar-Cederlof I, Plantin LO, et al: Albumin metabolism and gastrointestinal loss of protein in chronic renal failure. *Acta Med Scand* 201:353, 1977

8. Bernard DB: Metabolic abnormalities in nephrotic syndrome: Pathophysiology and complication, in Brenner BM, Stein JH (eds): *Nephrotic Syndrome*. New York, Churchill Livingstone, 1982, pp 85–120

9. Blahd WH, Fields M, Goldman R: The turnover rate of serum albumin in the nephrotic syndrome as determined by I^{131}-labeled albumin. *J Lab Clin Med* 46:747, 1955

10. Epstein AA: The nature and treatment of chronic parenchymatous nephritis (nephrosis). *JAMA* 69:444, 1971

11. Scott PJ, White BM, Winterbourn CC, et al: Low density lipoprotein peptide metabolism in nephrotic syndrome: A comparison with patterns observed in other syndromes characterized by hyperlipoproteinemia. *Aust Ann Med* 1:1, 1970

12. Marsh JB, Drabbin DL: Experimental reconstruction of the metabolic pattern of lipoid nephrosis: Key role of hepatic protein synthesis in hyperlipidemia. *Metabolism* 9:946, 1960

13. Rothschild MA, Oratz M, Wimer E, et al: Studies on albumin synthesis: The effects of dextran and cortisone on albumin metabolism in rabbits studied with albumin-I^{131}. *J Clin Invest* 40:545, 1961

14. Hyman LR, Wong PWK, Grossman A: Plasma lipoprotein lipase in children with idiopathic nephrotic syndrome. *Pediatrics* 44:1021, 1969

15. Kashyap ML, Strivastava LS, Hynd BA, et al: Apolipoprotein CII and lipoprotein lipase in human nephrotic syndrome. *Atherosclerosis* 35:29, 1980

16. Fielding CJ: Human lipoprotein lipase inhibition of acitivity by cholesterol. *Biochim Biophys Acta* 218:221, 1970

17. Cohen L, Cramp DG, Lewis AO, et al: The mechanism of hyperlipidaemia in nephrotic syndrome: Role of low albumin and the LCAT reaction. *Clin Chim Acta* 104:393, 1980

18. Dixit VM, Hettiaratchi ESG: The mechanism of hyperlipidemia in the nephrotic syndrome. *Med Hypotheses* 5:1327, 1979

19. Staprans I, Anderson CD, Lurz FW: Separation of a lipoprotein lipase co-factor from the α_1-acid glycoprotein fraction from the urine of nephrotic patients. *Biochim Biophys Acta* 617:514, 1980

20. Rosenman RH, Friedman M: In vivo studies of the role of albumin in nephrotic rats. *J Clin Invest* 39:700, 1957

21. Baxter JH, Goodman HC, Havel RJ: Serum lipid and lipoprotein alterations in nephrosis. *J Clin Invest* 39:455, 1960

22. Tall AR, Small DM: Plasma high density lipoproteins. *N Engl J Med* 299:1232, 1978

23. Felts JM, Mayerle JA, Urinary loss of plasma high density lipoproteins—a possible cause of the hyperlipidemia of the nephrotic syndrome. *Circulation* 50:265, 1974

24. Morris D, Trafford D, Makin H: High density lipoproteinuria in the nephrotic syndrome. *Clin Sci Mol Med* 53:5, 1977

25. Chopra JS, Mallick NP, Stone MC: Hyperlipoproteinemias in nephrotic syndrome. *Lancet* 1:317, 1971

26. Newmark SR, Anderson CF, Donadio JV, et al: Lipoprotein profiles in adult nephrotics. *Mayo Clin Proc* 50:359, 1975

27. Gherardi E, Rota E, Calandra S, et al: Relationship among the concentration of serum lipoproteins and changes in their chemical composition in patients with untreated nephrotic syndrome. *Eur J Clin Invest* 7:563, 1977
28. Mallick NP, Short CD: The nephrotic syndrome and ischemic heart disease. *Nephron* 27:54, 1981
29. Berlyne GM, Mallick NP: Ischemic heart disease as a complication of nephrotic syndrome. *Lancet* 2:399, 1969
30. Cameron JS, Wass V, Jarrett RJ, et al: Nephrotic syndrome and cardiovascular disease. *Lancet* 2:1017, 1979
31. Wass V, Cameron JS: Cardiovascular disease and the nephrotic syndrome: The other side of the coin. *Nephron* 27:58, 1981
32. Lopes-Virella M, Virella G, DeBeukelaev M, et al: Urinary high density lipoprotein in minimal change glomerular disease and chronic glomerulonephritis. *Clin Chim Acta* 94:73, 1979
33. Gordon T, Castelli WP, Hjortland MC, et al: High density lipoprotein as protection factor against coronary heart disease. *Am J Med* 62:707, 1977
34. Bridgman JF, Rosen SM, Throp JM: Complications during clofibrate treatment of nephrotic syndrome hyperlipoproteinaemia. *Lancet* 1:506, 1972
35. Cartwright GE, Gubler CJ, Wintrobe MM: Studies on copper metabolism. XI. Copper and iron metabolism in the nephrotic syndrome. *J Clin Invest* 33:685, 1954
36. Freeman RM, Richards CJ, Rames LK: Zinc metabolism in aminonucleoside induced nephrosis. *Am J Clin Nutr* 28:699, 1975
37. Ellis D: Anemia in the course of the nephrotic syndrome secondary to transferrin depletion. *J Pediatr* 90:953, 1977
38. Hancock FE, Onstad JW, Wolf PL: Transferrin loss into the urine with hypochromic, microcytic anemia. *Am J Clin Pathol* 65:73, 1976
39. Rifkind D, Kravetz HM, Knight V: Urinary excretion of iron-binding protein in the nephrotic syndrome. *N Engl J Med* 265:114, 1961
40. Reimold EW: Changes in zinc metabolism during the course of the nephrotic syndrome. *Am J Dis Child* 134:46, 1980
41. Feinstein EI, Kaptein EM, Nicoloff JT, et al: Thyroid function in patients with nephrotic syndrome and normal renal function. *Am J Nephrol* 2:70–76, 1982
42. Musa BU, Seal US, Doe RP: Excretion of corticosteroid-binding globulin, thyroxine-binding globulin and total protein in adult males with nephrosis: Effect of sex hormones. *J Clin Endocrinol* 27:768, 1967
43. Goldstein DA, Haldmann B, Sherman D: Vitamin D metabolites and calcium metabolism in patients with nephrotic syndrome and normal renal function. *J Clin Endocrinol Metab* 52:116, 1981
44. Barragry JM, France MW, Carter ND, et al: Vitamin D metabolism in nephrotic syndrome. *Lancet* 2:629, 1977
45. Schmidt-Gayk H, Schmitt W, Grawunder C: 25-Hydroxy-vitamin D in nephrotic syndrome. *Lancet* 2:105, 1977
46. Malluche HH, Goldstein DA, Massry SG: Osteomalacia and hyperparathyroid bone disease in patients with nephrotic syndrome. *J Clin Invest* 63:494, 1979
47. Goldstein DA, Oda Y, Kurokawa K, et al: Blood levels of 25-hydroxy-vitamin D in nephrotic syndrome. Studies in 26 patients. *Ann Intern Med* 87:664, 1977
48. Chan YL, Mason RS, Parmentier M, et al: Vitamin D metabolism in nephrotic rats. *Kidney Int* 24:336–341, 1983
49. Emerson K, Beckman WW: Calcium metabolism in nephrosis. I. A description of an

abnormality in calcium metabolism in children with nephrosis. *J Clin Invest* 24:564, 1945

50. Lim P, Jacob E, Chio LF, et al: Serum ionized calcium in nephrotic syndrome. *Q J Med* 45:421, 1976

51. Jones H, Peters DK, Morgan DB, et al: Observations on calcium metabolism in the nephrotic syndrome. *Q J Med* 36:301, 1967

52. Lim P, Jacob E, Took EPC, et al: Calcium and phosphorous metabolism in nephrotic syndrome. *Q J Med* 56:238, 1977

53. Llach F: Nephrotic syndrome: Hypercoagulability, renal vein thrombosis, and other thromboembolic complications, in Brenner BM, Stein JH (eds): *Nephrotic Syndrome*. New York, Churchill Livingstone, 1982, pp 121–144

54. Vaziri N: Nephrotic syndrome and coagulation and fibrinolytic abnormalities. *Am J Nephrol* 3:1–6, 1983

55. Kanfer A, Kleinknetch D, Broyer M, et al: Coagulation studies in 45 cases of nephrotic syndrome without uremia. *Thromb Diathes Haemorrh* 24:562, 1970

56. Kendall AG, Lohmann RE, Dossetor JB, et al: Nephrotic syndrome: A hypercoagulable state. *Arch Intern Med* 127:1021, 1971

57. Bang N, Trygstad C, Schroeder J, et al: Enhanced platelet function in glomerular renal disease. *J Lab Clin Med* 81:651, 1973

58. Kauffman R, Veltkamp J, Tilberg N, et al: Acquired antithrombin III deficiency and thrombosis in the nephrotic syndrome. *Am J Med* 65:607, 1978

59. Andrassy K, Ritz E, Bommer J: Hypercoagulability in the nephrotic syndrome. *Klin Wochenschr* 58:1029, 1980

60. Handley DA, Lawrence JR: Factor IX deficiency in the nephrotic syndrome. *Lancet* 1:1079, 1967

61. Green D, Arruda J, Honig G, et al: Urinary loss of clotting factor due to hereditary membranous nephropathy. *Am J Clin Pathol* 65:376, 1976

62. Rayer PFO: *Traite des Maladies des Reims et des Alterations de la Secretions Urinaire*, vol 2. Paris, JB Baillière, 1840, pp 590–599

63. Llach F, Koffler A, Finick E, et al: On the incidence of renal vein thrombosis in the nephrotic syndrome. *Arch Intern Med* 137:333, 1977

64. Klassen J, Sugisaki T, Milgrom F, et al: Studies of multiple renal lesions in Heymann nephritis. *Lab Invest* 25:577, 1971

65. Llach F, Papper S, Massry SG: The clinical spectrum of renal vein thrombosis: Acute and chronic. *Am J Med* 69:819, 1981

66. Peterson PA, Berggard I: Urinary immunoglobulin components in normal, tubular and glomerular proteinuria. *Eur J Clin Invest* 1:255, 1971

67. Waldmann TA, Strober W, Mogielnicki RP: The renal handling of low molecular weight proteins. II. Disorders of serum protein catabolism in patients with tubular proteinuria. The nephrotic syndrome in uremia. *J Clin Invest* 51:2162, 1972

68. Ooi BS, Ooi YM, Hsu A, et al: Diminished synthesis of immunoglobulin by lymphocytes of patients with idiopathic membranous glomerulopathy. *J Clin Invest* 65:787–797, 1980

69. Shakib F, Hardwicke J, Stanworth DR: Asymmetric depression in the serum level of IgG subclasses in patients with nephrotic syndrome. *Clin Exp Immunol* 28:506, 1977

70. Giangiacomo J, Cleary TG, Cole BR, et al: Serum immunoglobulins in the nephrotic syndrome. A possible cause of minimal change nephrotic syndrome. *N Engl J Med* 293:8, 1975

71. Groshong T, Mendelson L, Mendoza S, et al: Serum IgE in patients with minimal change nephrotic syndrome. *J Pediatr* 83:767, 1973

72. Sissons J, Woodrow D, Curtis JR, et al: Isolated glomerulonephritis with IgA deposits. *Br Med J* 3:611, 1975
73. Lewis EJ, Carpenter CB, Schur PH: Serum complement component levels in human glomerulonephritis. *Ann Intern Med* 75:555, 1971
74. McLean RH, Forsgren A, Bjorkstein B, et al: Decreased serum factor B concentration associated with decreased opsonization of *Escherichia coli* in the idiopathic nephrotic syndrome. *Petiatr Res* 11:910, 1977
75. Mallick NP, Williams RJ, McFarlane H, et al: Cell-mediated immunity in nephrotic syndrome. *Lancet* 1:507–509, 1972
76. Mallick NP: The pthogenesis of minimal change nephropathy. *Clin Nephrol* 7:87, 1977
77. Llach F: *Renal Vein Thrombosis*. New York, Futura Publishing Co., 1983

12

Clinical Proteinuria

GEORGE E. SCHREINER

INTRODUCTION

Proteinuria is a major screening pointer for the nephrologist. It may be detected in mass surveys, initial or annual physical examinations, school, employment, insurance, or military examinations, office and hospital admission routines, or even by foam in the urinal. Hippocrates said, "Bubbles on the surface of the urine are a sign of disease of the kidneys...." Whatever the mode of discovery, proteinuria is a call for action. *Res ipsa loquitur*; proteinuria speaks. It demands further workup, laboratory testing, or referral to a nephrologist.

Proteinuria has many causes, which are outlined in Table I. These vary in complexity as does our degree of understanding. Disruption of capillary continuity by endothelial swelling, proliferation, capillary necrosis, thromboses, or fat emboli provide a plausible morphologic explanation for proteinuria. It is usually accompanied by cells of varied types in the urinary sediment. Permselectivity changes may occur with proteins of smaller size (e.g., Bence Jones) or longer shapes (eliptical versus spheroid). More recently, our knowledge has been extended by attention to both the electrostatic charges in potentially filterable molecules and the negative charge on the glycoprotein and sialoprotein components of layers in the basement membrane.

Tubular proteinuria of massive proportions is rare but can occur when the extensive peritubular capillary plexus is injured and stripped of the usually efficient epithelial cell barrier. An example is described below in depth. Tubular proteinuria of lesser severity (usually less than 2.5 g/day) may be seen during the development phase of acute tubular necrosis whether by nephrotoxins, ischemia, vasoconstriction, acute and subacute rejection syndromes in kidney transplantation, Wilson's dis-

GEORGE E. SCHREINER • Department of Medicine, Division of Nephrology, Georgetown University School of Medicine, Washington, D.C. 20007.

Table I. Proteinuria:
Classification of Causes

Glomerular
  Disease → morphologic changes
  Permselectivity physiolgical change
    Size
    Shape
    Surface charge
Tubular
  Capillary leak—ATN
  ↓Reabsorption
  MADE—(T-H, cadmium)
  Tubulointerstitial disease
Hemodynamic
  Vasoconstrictive
    Catechols
    Angiotensin
  Congestive
    Heart failure
    Renal venous obstruction
  ↑Filtered load
  Diuretic
  Febrile
Lower urinary tract
  Prostate, bladder
  Semen, s. vesicle
Transient
  Exercise
  Psychosomatic stress
Postural
  True orthostatic
  Postural component
  Lymphatic

---

ease, Fanconi syndrome, Balkan nephropathy, severe hypokalemia with potassium depletion, and drug nephrotoxicity. Some of the major drugs associated with acute hypersensitivity interstitial nephritis are shown in Table II.

Decreased tubular reabsorption of filtered protein has often been proposed but seldom established for a chemical transport process and is unlikely to account for more than 3–7 g of albumin in a 24-h collection. Tamm–Horsfall protein was discovered in the 1920s and is still without a meaningful role. We hypothesize its use as a packaging material. By forming the outer matrix of granular casts, it may protect sensitive brush-border elements and intraluminal membranes from the irritating effects

Table II. Drugs Associated with Acute Hypersensitivity Interstitial Nephritis

Cyclosporine A	NSAIDS
Penicillins	Allopurinol
(Naphcillin, Ampicillin)	
Sulfonamide	Antipyrine
Polymyxins	Azathioprine
Rifampin	Gold
Cephalosporins	Phenylbutazone
Cotrimoxazole	Phenazone
Bismuth	Phenindione
para-Aminosalicylate	Phenytoin
Thiazides	Gelafenine
Furosemide	Erythromycin

of protein aggregates such as myoglobin, light chains, and globulin fractions. One of the differentiating features of tubulointerstitial disease clinically has been proteinuria of less than 1 g/day. However, some exceptions to this rule appear to be emerging. Both Kincaid-Smith and Nanra[1] have reported proteinuria greater than 1 g in a small fraction of patients with analgesic nephropathy, a predominantly interstitial disease. It is not clear whether there is a constant association in these patients between high proteinuria and focal sclerosis of the glomeruli. Another possible exception is uric acid nephropathy, which is discussed below.

Less dynamic considerations have been invoked to explain febrile proteinuria (e.g., using a Kettering hypertherm), stress proteinuria (e.g., venipuncture for venereal disease testing), some exercise and postural proteinurias, and the known enhancement of permeability by agents such as norepinephrine and angiotensin. Increased venous pressure from plethora, rapid volume expansion, congestive heart failure, tricuspid insufficiency, and renal-vein thrombosis has been classically attributed to dilatation of renal venules and possible enhancement of lymphatic flow by a change in Starling forces. Augmentation of renal proteinuria occurs in both water and solute diuresis.

Clinically, one must be very careful to properly diagnose protein emanating from the lower urinary tract including secretions from prostate, testes, seminal vesicles, anomalous remnants, bladder diverticuli, vesicular inflammation, tumors, etc. I have seen many an insurance policy refused because of urinalysis after intercourse, nocturnal emissions, barium enemas, sigmoidoscopy, or even simple rectal examinations.

Transient proteinuria has been described in the literature under such terms as "benign," "intermittent," "muscular," "exercise," "march" (army term), "physiological," and "idiopathic." It is extremely frequent in children on initial pediatric workups. Its significance is usually determined simply by repetitive examination.

Postural proteinuria may be transient or fixed. It also may be pure or represent an augmentation of already elevated levels of protein excretion. We have found it useful to define "postural component" as measured rate of less than 0.1 mg/min in the horizontal position with a sustained increment of fourfold or more in the upright posture. Most of our potentially serious biopsy findings have been in the postural component group so defined. One study of fixed orthostatic proteinuria[2] found 45% subtle glomerular alteration but a good prognosis for renal function in a 10-year follow-up study.

CLINICAL METHODOLOGY

There are many convenient techniques for obtaining a semiquantitative estimate of protein excretion on a fresh urine sample. They should always be accompanied by a measurement of osmolality or specific gravity since urinary dilution may mask a clinically significant proteinuria. The flocculation method is usually done by heating urine and adding glacial acetic acid. False positives are rendered by iodides, contrast agents, penicillins, and metabolites of tolbutamide. The precipitation tests employ sulfosalicylic acid or nitric acid with grading of the turbidity. There are some false positives including concentrated uric acid in a newborn. These methods can detect 5–10 mg/dl. "Dipsticks" have impregnated paper with an indicator, tetrabromephenol blue, calibrated to a color chart of pH 3.0. Protein changes the pH in proportion to its concentration and is readable from a color chart. False positives may be rendered by highly alkaline urine. Dipsticks are sensitive only down to 30 mg/dl and may be negative with dilute urine. They are insensitive to light chains. Quantitative proteinuria is often measured on a timed sample (usually 12- or 24-h urine) by precipitation techniques by using sulfosalicylic acid, phosphotungstic acid, Esbach's picric acid–citric acid reagent, or Tsuchiya's reagent with a calibrated tube or by a turbidity method and nephelometer or a biochemical method and colorimeter. Urine electrophoresis is used when light chains are expected in the urine. The monoclonal spike may be seen in most patients with myeloma. The electrophoretic pattern may be used as a fast clinical estimate of selectivity.

FUNCTIONAL CONSIDERATIONS

About 12 g of plasma proteins traverse the glomerular capillaries in a day. Most of this is effectively retained by the membrane barrier. Albumin has a negative charge at body pH and is less permeable than neutral or cationic molecules of similar size. Increased permeability has been demonstrated by manipulation of the sialo protein and glycosaminoglycan anionic residues, which impede the movement of negatively charged macromolecules. Normal protein excretion rates are up to 0.1 mg/min, slightly greater in women than men. Sixty percent of this by weight consists of albumin (40%), fragments of immunoglobulins, enzymes, hormones, and other protein; IgG represents 5–10%, light chains 5%, and IgA 3%; IgM and IgD are rarely detectable. The residual 40% consists of Tamm–Horsfall mucoprotein, proteins derived from epithelial cells and the urogenital tract. In the early 1950s, the late Leonard Berman and I[3] measured quantitative proteinuria in 50 consecutive patients admitted to hospital with nephrotic syndrome.

This study was extended to 184 patients with frequently encountered renal diseases. It was determined that nonnephrotic organic renal diseases usually had less than 2 g of protein per $1.73m^2$ per day, whereas most nephrotic syndrome patients had excretion rates above 3 to 3.5 g/day.

Continued experience with thousands of quantitative protein determinations has verified the bimodal distribution curve of clinical proteinuria, with a very small percentage of patients falling into the 2- to 3-g range. Even some of these, when followed sequentially, are found to be either on their way into or out of a nephrotic syndrome. This quantitative notion of glomerular permeability has now been widely incorporated into the definition of the nephrotic syndrome[4] and appears in most modern textbooks.

A permeability index accounts for the major variables in quantitative protein excretion and allows one to compare individuals with markedly different body surface areas, filtration rates, and plasma albumin concentrations. More importantly, it provides a convenient method of following the serial progress of patients who have a morphological lesion producing significant proteinuria. If, for example, a patient is seen in the clinic with 20 g of proteinuria and a GFR of 100 ml/min and then returns a year later with a proteinuria of 15 g/day and a GFR of 50 ml/min, our favorite question becomes "Is the patient better or worse?" From the standpoint of metabolism, the patient may be better off since, with a good diet, his liver can more easily synthesize 15 g a day than 20 g. However, from the standpoint of the kidney lesion, he is worse, for he has halved his filtration rate but only quartered his proteinuria. This descrepancy is compatible with extension of the lesion to a previously uninvolved capillary filtration surface.

Hardwicke[5] introduced the concept of selectivity in the consideration of proteinuria when they found a differential clearance of α_1-mucoprotein equal to 124% of the albumin clearance and a β-globulin of 29%, γ-globulin 27%, and the α_{II}-globulin 13% of the albumin clearance. When the slope K was measured in various diseases in 60 patients, it became obvious that lipoid nephrosis possesses the highest level of selectivity.

THE FATE OF FILTERED PROTEIN

The conditions for gel formation (acidification plus concentration) exist in the nephron beginning at the distal portion of the convoluted tubule. Some years ago, Rutecki, in our laboratory, pursued an attempt to delineate the nature of the granules often found in the granular casts associated with so-called "wide-open" nephrotic syndrome in which proteinuria is quite massive. This was done by making antibodies against all of the common serum proteins and coupling them with fluorescein. Serum proteins always appeared in the granular aggregates or the core of the cast. In addition, we used C-reactive protein and antibodies against Tamm–Horsfall protein and suitable reagent controls. The outer matrix of casts was found to consist of Tamm–Horsfall protein, and all of the serum proteins could be found in the granules.

SPECIAL CONSIDERATIONS IN TUBULAR PROTEINURIA

Although massive proteinuria continues to be a clinically useful differentiation between primary glomerular and primary tubular disease, there are some special exceptions to this rule, and, fortunately, the mechanisms are better understood. The first mechansim, briefly noted above, is the dual lesion of peritubular capillary permeability coupled with the functional loss of the epithelial cell barrier. This is illustrated by the following case:

> H.N. was a 24-year-old black male with a primary diagnosis of nephroscle-rosis who had a living-donor transplant with a two-antigen match performed 2 months following a nephrectomy of his own end-stage kidneys. The sur-

gery was followed by 4 h of oliguria with subsequent beginning of diuresis. One hundred fifty rads of radiation was administered to the graft on post-transplant days 1,2,4, and 5. The transplant continued to diurese, the plasma creatinine declined to 1.1, and he was measured to have 1.0 g of proteinuria. On posttransplant day 11, he had an acute rejection, which was reversed by standard pulse therapy. On day 28 he rejected again; on day 29 a scan showed good flow in the graft. On day 33 an intravenous pyelogram was done, and another 150 rads was administered to the transplant. On day 37 an arteriogram was done, which was followed by oliguria to day 43 and diagnosed as a nephrotoxic acute tubular necrosis, possibly caused by both contrast agent and radiation. Proteinuria was measured at 38 g/24 h on day 45. Biopsies were done on the transplant on days 34 and 56. Capillaries can be found along the tubules demonstrating actual leakage of protein including fibrinogen. We believe that this illustrates tubular proteinuria in the nephrotic range. It should be especially noted that the proteinuria rose when the GFR fell and fell when the GFR rose. This is directly opposite the usual clinical experience with glomerular lesions leading to massive proteinuria. The clinical evolution in such cases usually shows a rise in proteinuria at least in the early phase of increase in the glomerular filtration rate. No foot process fusion was present.

A second mechanism that should be considered when the nephrotic-range proteinuria accompanies an otherwise predominately tubular or interstitial disease is the potential for concomitant development of focal glomerulosclerosis. Recent data have been presented to indicate a very significant relationship between the quantity of proteinuria and the duration of proteinuria before the development of end-stage kidney disease with irreversible loss of kidney function. There are also a number of experimental models that have given insights into the pathophysiology of focal sclerosis (Table III). With the lesion of focal sclerosis occurring in so many varied disease situations, no clear-cut pathogenesis has been worked out. Some of the possibilities that could be suggested are: (1) local immune injury with a release of a substance that is locally cytotoxic to epithelial tissue; (2) the possibility that in the presence of proteinuria a cellular toxin could be carried on a protein molecule through the basement membrane to injure one or a group of epithelial cells; (3) that fo-

Table III. Proteinuria: Focal Glomerular Sclerosis

Experimental models
1. Aminonucleoside
2. N.N.-Diacetylbenzidine
3. Aging Rat
4. ↓Renal Mass
5. Overload Proteinuria

cal sclerosis represents a late stage of focal proliferative disease or (4) is a result of hypertension; (5) the result of therapy with steroids and immunosuppressives; and (6) that those cases of lipoid nephrosis complicated by focal sclerosis represent a separate disease from the onset; (7) focal sclerosis engrafted on an otherwise interstitial disease may produce a significant proteinuria, which, although it is usually in the 1- to 3-g range, may rise into the nephrotic range with or without the clinical features of nephrotic syndrome. In the clearly interstitial diseases such as analgesic nephropathy, it is extremely rare to see a proteinuria above 10 g per day without renal vein thrombosis. When it is high, the course of deteriorated function appears to be accelerated, and in a relatively short interval function of the kidney will be lost.

PROTEINURIA IN GOUTY NEPHROPATHY

Because of anecdotal reports that gout *per se* or uric acid nephropathy could produce nephrotic-range proteinuria, we had a retrospective chart review of 82 patients selected from our files of diagnostic patients who had a strong history of gouty arthritis (usually chronic and recurrent) or proven uric acid stones or both and qualitative proteinuria at the time of hospital admission; 19 patients or 23% had a measured 24-h urine in excess of 1 g/24 h. There were 17 males and two females; five blacks, 13 caucasians, and one oriental. The mean age was 47, the median 46. The mean highest serum uric acid was 9.3, the median 8.8 (range 6.2–18.9). The mean highest measured urinary 24-h protein was 3.9 g/day, the median 2.6 (range 1.2–12.6). Only two patients had normal filtration rates. The mean endogenous creatinine clearance was 41, the median 37.

Only two patients exceeded 7 g/24 h of proteinuria. One (11 g/day) had a previous partial cystectomy for carcinoma of the bladder (negative for cancer at time of our study), and the other (12.6 g) had a clinically full nephrotic syndrome and biopsy-proven membranous glomerulonephritis. Many of these patients had potential causes other then gouty kidney for their proteinuria, e.g., diabetes (2), polycystic disease (2), medullary cystic disease (1), hypertension (9), and congestive heart failure (several).

Our impression from this brief study is that even in severe gouty patients requiring hospitalization with substantial defects in renal function, massive proteinuria is uncommon. More often than not, other substantive conditions are present that may offer a better explanation for heavy proteinuria then gouty nephropathy *per se*. Gouty nephropathy thus seems to conform to the general clinical rules of tubulointerstitial nephritis.

THERAPEUTIC CONSIDERATIONS

It is beyond the scope of this paper to discuss in detail the therapy of the nephrotic syndrome as a cause of massive proteinuria. When such proteinuria is caused by identified nephroallergens (e.g., RHUS toxin), it should be avoided or withdrawn; when it is caused by infection (e.g., malaria or shunt nephritis), the treatment of the primary infection will often produce a remission. When it is caused by a drug, the offending molecule should be withheld. When it is idiopathic, the mainstay of therapy continues to be high-protein diet, steroids, and immunosuppressive drugs. When proteinuria is unresponsive to any of these methods and is of such a magnitude that it is impossible for the liver to synthesize enough albumin to stay in nitrogen balance, then severe malnutrition and muscle and tissue wasting will result. At such a time, a good glomerular filtration rate becomes, in a sense, an enemy. There have been a number of heroic measures suggested for therapeutic intervention to spare protein loss. These cases are so rare that no truly prospective studies can be done. The heroic measures have included reduction of the glomerular filtration rate by prostaglandin synthetase inhibitors such as indomethacin; unilateral nephrectomy, medical nephrectomy by shredded absorbable gelatin sponge administered through a catheter; medical nephrectomy by mercury salts injected intramuscularly (see M.M. Avram, this volume), selective injections of polymers that form an occlusive intraarterial mass, and, of course, bilateral nephrectomy followed by dialysis and/or transplantation.

ACKNOWLEDGMENTS. I wish to acknowledge the special help given by my editorial assistant, Mrs. Betty Mendelson, and also to express gratitude to the many patients who have permitted and supported clinical studies.

REFERENCES

1. Kincaid-Smith P, Nanva RS: Personal communication
2. Thompson AL, Durrett RR, Robinson RR: Fixed and reproducible orthostatic proteinuria. *Ann Int Med* 73: 235, 1970
3. Berman LB, Schreiner GE: Clinical and histiolgic spectrum of nephrotic sydrome. *Am J Med* 24: 249, 1958
4. Glassock RS: The nephrotic syndrome. *Hosp Pract* 14:105, 1979
5. Hardwicke J: Serum and urine protein changes in the nephrotic sydrome. *Proc Roy Soc Med* 47:834, 1954
6. Rutecki GJ, Goldsmith C, Schreiner GE: Characterization of proteins in urinary casts: Fluorescent antibody identification of Tamm-Horsfall mucoprotein in matrix and serum proteins in granules. *N Engl J Med* 284: 1049, 1971

Part IV

Expectant or Aggressive Management

Proteinuria, although widely treated, still presents the clinician with a dilemma of its "effective" treatability. Protein leakage into urine can be reduced by altering physiological forces as demonstrated by Berlyne and associates, who raised interstitial pressure by the unique approach of placing the nephrotic patient in water. They describe 11 adults with the nephrotic syndrome of various etiologies who were immersed in tepid water to their necks. Water immersion resulted in a sharp water diuresis and a hypotonic urine. A clinical application of water immersion has yet to be devised, although its potential in diverse edematous conditions is evident.

Porush, in a skillful, scholarly analysis, next addresses the difficult topic of how and when to limit or reverse proteinuria in idiopathic membranous glomerulopathy using corticosteroids and cytotoxic drugs. Although a collaborative trial of short-term steroids in nonazotemic patients appeared to show steroid-induced improvement, the results were far from spectacular, leaving the clinician uneasy over how best to manage proteinuria in membranous glomerulopathy, which will probably turn out to be a family of diseases.

Persistent, massive proteinuria can become life endangering. Hypotension evolving into shock may be the consequence of total loss of oncotic pressure in extreme hypoalbuminemia. Avram reports his unusual response to imminent death from protein loss in what he terms a "malignant porteinuria" syndrome (over 25 g/day) by using the new medical approach of destruction of glomerular but not renal endocrine function (medical nephrectomy). With several glomerular diseases, especially advanced focal sclerosis, transglomerular passage of proteins can be enormously increased, saturating the capacity of renal tubules to take up filtered protein; urinary protein excretion then reaches massive proportions. To selectively destroy renal function, Avram used parenteral sodium mercaptomerin, a mercurial diuretic, which promptly abated glomerular filtration in two patients who, despite irreversible uremia, continued to have massive, life-threatening protein loss. Therapy was successful in that protein loss stopped abruptly and plasma volume was restored. Other renal toxins capable of being employed for producing medical nephrectomy are reviewed.

Kiley, Case, and Bower next confirm that medical nephrectomy for malignant proteinuria was rational and workable in a patient with focal sclerosis on dialysis. Finally, Doolan recounts his use of medical nephrectomy in a uremic diabetic with proteinuria.

Given the need to destroy rather than preserve kidneys in uremia with persistent protein loss, the derivative question arises: "Would medical nephrectomy for nephrosis ever be appropriate when sufficient renal function to sustain life remains?" Although this question remains to be answered, medical nephrectomy for dialysis patients suffering with "malignant proteinuria" appears to be an effective new treatment modality.

M.M.A.

13

Water Immersion
in Nephrotic Syndrome

J. SUTTON, D. E. BROWN, A. J. ADLER, J. E. RUBIN,
M. SEIDMAN, E. A. FRIEDMAN, AND G. M. BERLYNE

INTRODUCTION

Water immersion up to the neck has been described in detail in a series of papers by Epstein and his colleagues dealing with the response in the normal subject and in the cirrhotic patient.[1-4] Epstein concluded that water immersion in 4 ft of water resulted in a physiological response similar to that produced by the rapid intravenous infusion of 2 liters of saline and that there was central venous distention with fluid compressed out of the lower limbs and abdomen into the central veins. These mechanisms have been discussed at length by Epstein and his colleagues in the normal and in the cirrhotic. However, an analogous situation, the response in the nephrotic patient, was ignored until we investigated the response to water immersion in 11 nephrotics.[5-8]

The group of 11 nephrotics consisted of eight males and three females aged 17 to 64 years: four had membranous glomerulopathy, two had lipid nephrosis, one had interstitial nephitis, three had focal glomerulosclerosis, and one had diabetic glomerulosclerosis. All patients were on a 50-mEq Na diet, and frusemide had been stopped 3–7 days before the test. Prednisone had been discontinued 1 week prior to the study. All patients had control urine collections from 9 a.m. to 4 p.m. either the day before immersion or one week later. They had free fluid intake, drinking according to thirst.

On the day of immersion, an intravenous inulin loading dose was

J. SUTTON, D. E. BROWN, A. J. ADLER, J. E. RUBIN, M. SEIDMAN, E. A. FRIEDMAN, AND G. M. BERLYNE • Department of Medicine, Brooklyn Veterans Administration Medical Center and State University of New York Downstate Medical Center, Brooklyn, New York 11203.

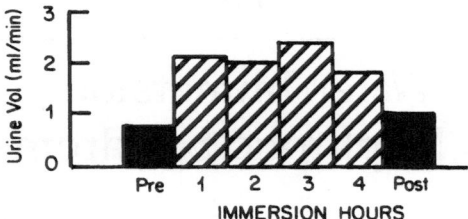

Figure 1. Urine volume increased significantly on immersion (median values given). Preimmersion control versus third hour of immersion ($P < 0.005$).

started at 9 a.m.; and infusion after 60 min of equilibration, urine and plasma collections were made at hourly intervals. After a 1-h period seated by the bath, the so-called preimmersion period, the patient was immersed, seated, up to the neck in 4 feet of water at 34°C. Each hour the patients were removed from the water, toweled dry, passed urine spontaneously, and had a blood sample taken. They then went back into the bath. Total time of immersion was 4 h. After this, they spent a further hour seated—the "postimmersion hour."

Chemical methods for creatinine, urea, uric acid, chloride, and phosphate were standard Technicon Auto Analyzer methods carried out on an Auto Analyzer II; those for sodium and potassium were by IL flame photometer, Model 343; tests for calcium and magnesium were by means of atomic absorption flame photometry using an IL atomic absorpsion instrument Model 251 (Instrumentation Labs, Inc., Lexington, MA).

RESULTS

Urine volume increased rapidly and significantly with water immersion; this correlated with a mean weight loss of 2.4 kg during the immersion period (Fig. 1).

Urine osmolality fell to a median value of 220 mOsm/kg in the first

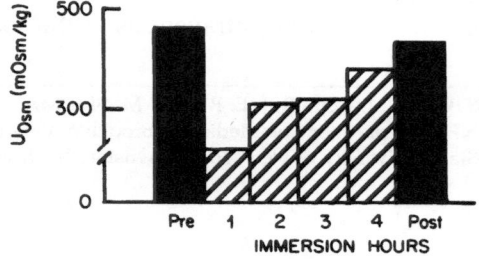

Figure 2. Urine osmolality fell significantly to a median value of 220 mOsm/kg in first hour from 475 mOsm/kg ($P < 0.001$).

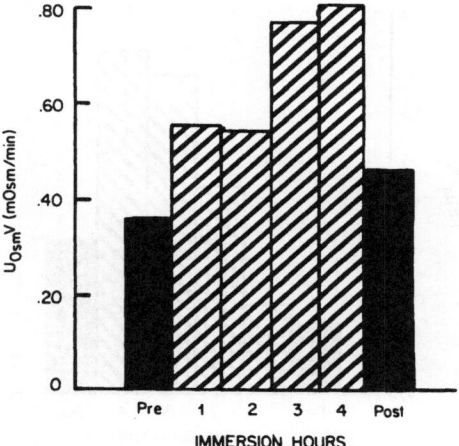

Figure 3. Osmolar excretion increased significantly on immersion, reaching a maximum in the fourth hour of immersion ($P < 0.04$).

hour of immersion and slowly increased during the subsequent 3 h of immersion. It rose to 438 mOsm/kg in the postimmersion hour (Fig. 2).

Urine osmolar excretion increased rapidly on immersion to a maximum of 0.81mOsm/min and fell to 0.44mOsm/min in the postimmersion hour (Fig. 3).

Urine sodium excretion rose fivefold during immersion when compared with control values (Fig. 4). FE_{Na} rose threefold by the fourth

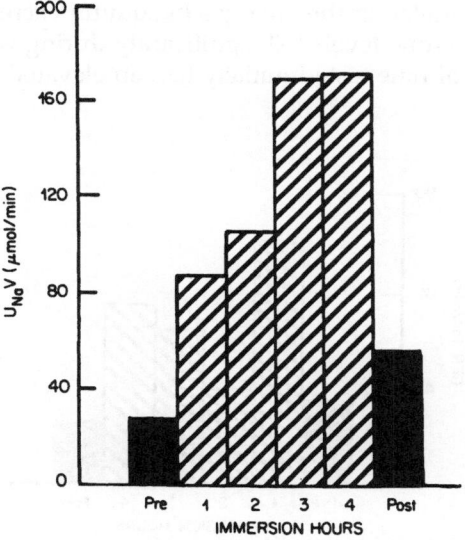

Figure 4. Sodium excretion rate rose significantly from a median value of 2.63 μmol/min to a maximum of 173.1 μmol/min ($P < 0.0025$).

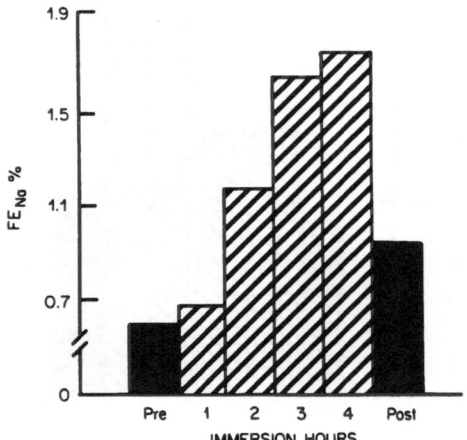

Figure 5. Fractional excretion of sodium increased significantly on immersion by second, third, and fourth hours ($P < 0.005$).

hour of immersion (Fig. 5). The slowness of the initial rise in FE_{Na} when compared with sodium excretion may be explained by the rapid rise in GFR in the first hour of immersion, which increased the denominator in the expression $FE = C_{Na}/C_{inulin}$ (Fig. 6).

Potassium excretion ($U_K V$) doubled on immersion, but fractional excretion of potassium did not increase significantly.

Urine chloride excretion and FE_{Cl} increased significantly during water immersion, paralleling the changes in sodium excretion (Figs. 7, 8).

Plasma aldosterone levels fell significantly during water immersion, but only two out of nine tested initially had an elevated plasma aldosterone level.

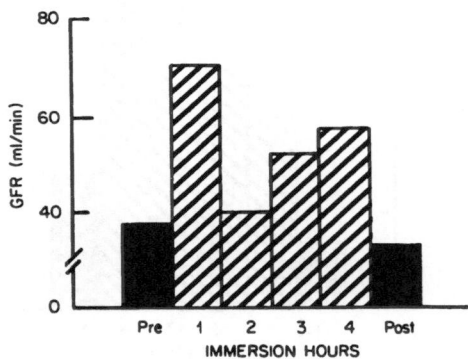

Figure 6. The GFR increased significantly in the first hour of immersion ($P < 0.01$). Overall, immersion GFR was not significantly different from pre- and postimmersion values.

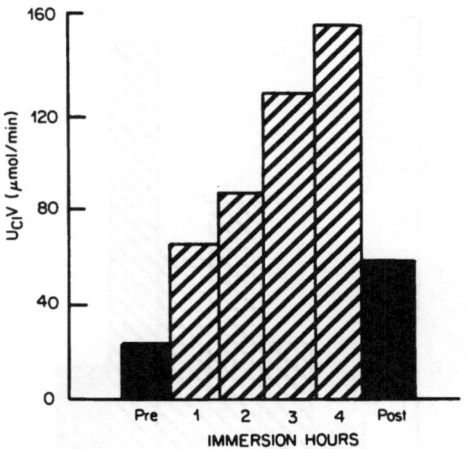

Figure 7. Chloride excretion rate rose significantly on immersion ($P < 0.0025$).

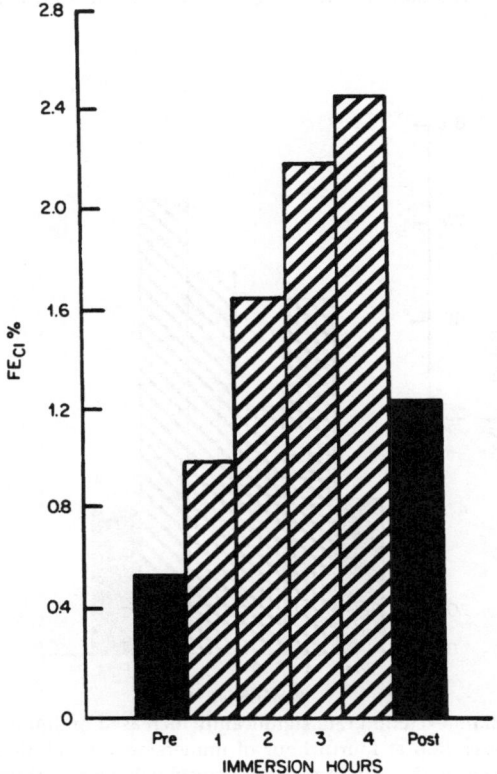

Figure 8. Fractional excretion of chloride rose significantly on immersion ($P < 0.005$).

J. Sutton *et al.*

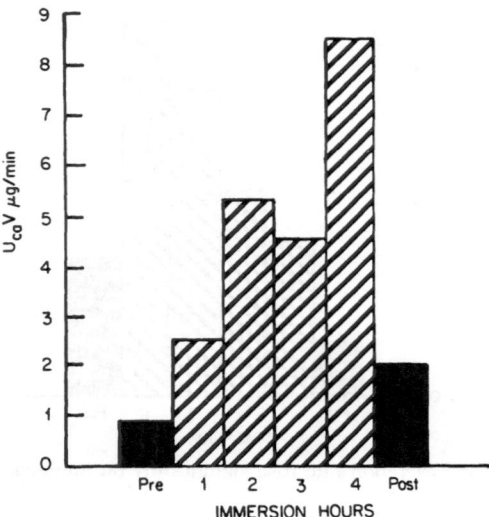

Figure 9. Calcium excretion rate rose significantly by the fourth hour of immersion
($2P < 0.02$).

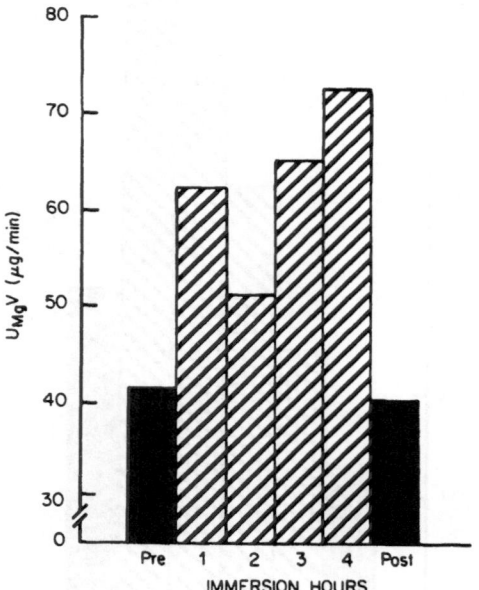

Figure 10. Magnesium excretion rate significantly increased on immersion ($P < 0.05$). Median magnesium excretion at fourth hour of immersion was 8.6 times higher than corresponding calcium excretion. Preimmersion control value was 206 times higher than calcium excretion at the same period.

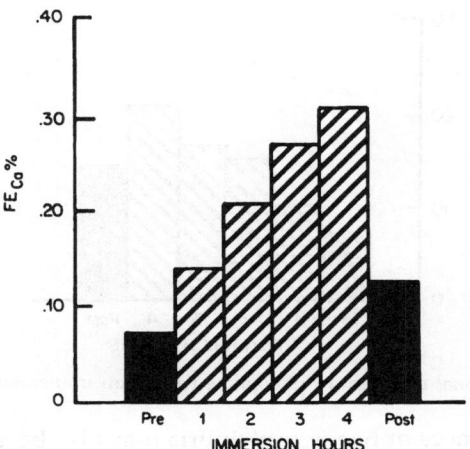

Figure 11. Fractional excretion of calcium rose from a median preimmersion control rate of 0.07% to a fourth-hour peak of 0.31% ($2P < 0.01$).

Urinary calcium excretion increased ninefold during water immersion. In three out of 11 patients, urine calcium excretion was minimal, less that $0.5\mu g$/min. In contrast, urinary magnesium was at least ten times greater and increased significantly during water immersion (Figs. 9, 10).

FE_{Ca} rose fivefold to 0.305% during immersion, whereas FE_{Mg} doubled on immersion and reached 10%, i.e., 30 times greater than simultaneous values of FE_{Ca} (Fig. 11).

Renal phosphate excretion more than doubled during water immersion (Fig. 12); FE_{PO_4} tripled during immersion (Fig. 13). T_mPO_4/GFR, calculated from the Watson–Bijvoet nomogram, was not significantly changed by immersion. The application of the Watson–Bijvoet nomogram is not strictly applicable to situations in which the GFR is below 40

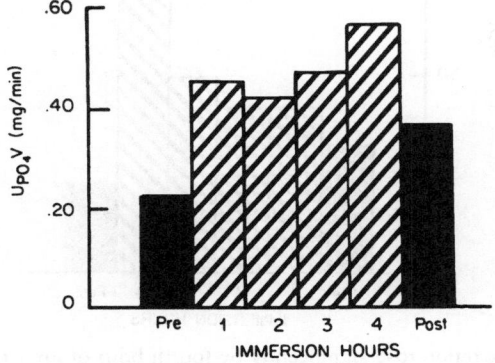

Figure 12. Phosphate excretion doubled by the fourth hour of immersion ($2P < 0.02$).

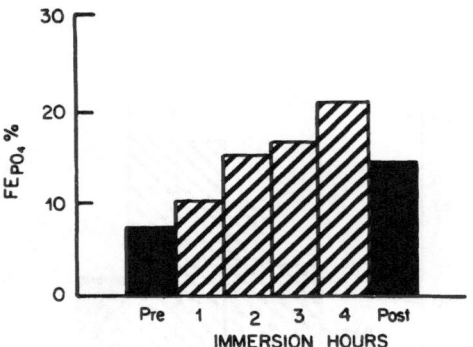

Figure 13. Fractional excretion of phosphate tripled on immersion ($2P < 0.01$).

ml/min; the presenece of heavy proteinuria may also be a confusing factor negating use of the nomogram in this particular circumstance.

Parathyroid hormone levels overall did not change on immersion. Although significant transient increases in PTH levels were observed during water immersion, these were insufficient to explain the increase in FE_{PO4}.

Urate excretion increased significantly from 0.38 mg/min before immersion to 0.62 mg/min in the fourth hour of immersion (Fig. 14). It decreased to 0.28 mg/min, falling below control values in the postimmersion hour. Fractional excretion of urate (*FE* urate) increased by 50% during water immersion (Fig. 15).

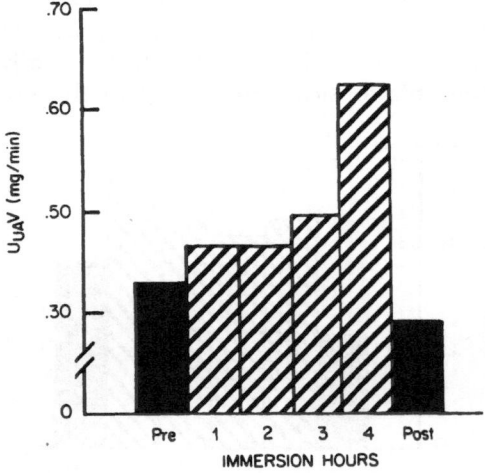

Figure 14. Urate excretion rose significantly by fourth hour of immersion ($P < 0.0125$).

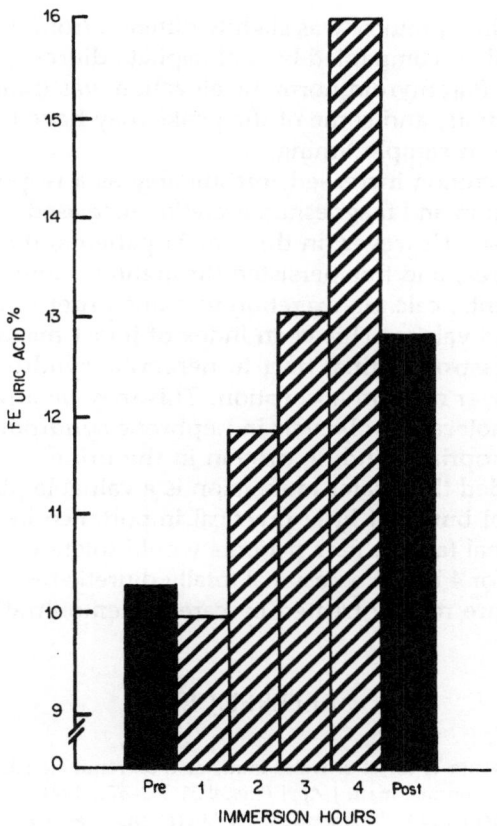

Figure 15. Fractional excretion rate of urate rose from a median value of 10.25% to a maximum value of 15.98% by the fourth hour of immersion ($P < 0.025$).

DISCUSSION

Epstein has pointed out that water immersion up to the neck causes, in the normal man, physiological responses akin to those of a rapid intravenous infusion of saline. This would be expected to result in a sodium chloride, phosphate, uric acid, calcium, and magnesium diuresis. The initial water diuresis is caused by and associated with an experimentally demonstrable fall in ADH secretion, the reason for which is unclear. Isotonic volume expansion is not usually associated with a fall in ADH secretion or with a water diuresis.

Phosphate diuresis has not been observed by Epstein *et al.* in normals and cirrhotics. We cannot offer explanations of the discrepancy in the nephrotic. Their protocol was slightly different from ours, but sodium diuresis is usually accompanied by a phosphate diuresis during isotonic ECF expansion. Parathyroid hormone elevation was transient, but PTH is secreted in bursts, and some of the peaks may have been missed because of chance in sample timing.

Uric acid excretion increased, presumably as a response to volume expansion. Calcium and magnesium excretion increased as expected with a sodium diuresis. However, in three of 11 patients, the urine was virtually calcium-free, and this persisted throughout immersion. In all the remaining patients, calcium excretion was one order of magnitude less than magnesium values. This is an index of intact magnesium absorption from the gastrointestinal tract in nephrotic syndrome when compared to the lower calcium absorption. This may be a reflection of the lower 25-OH cholecalciferol levels in nephrotic syndrome as a result of the loss of appropriate binding protein in the urine.

It is concluded that water immersion is a valuable physiopathological research tool but is of little practical importance in the day-to-day treatment of renal failure. Few patients would tolerate daily immersion up to the neck for 4 h; the occasional totally diuretic-resistant patient can have edema more readily treated by careful hemofiltration.

REFERENCES

1. Epstein M M, Saruta T: Effect of water immersion on renin aldosterone and renal sodium handling in normal man. *J Appl Physiol* 31:363–374, 1971
2. Epstein M, Schneider N S, Vaamonde C A: Alterations in acid–base homeostasis during water immersion in normal man. *J Lab Clin Med* 84:777–790, 1974
3. Epstein M: Cardiovascular and renal effects of head out immerison in man. *Circ Res* 39:620–628, 1976
4. Epstein M, Pins D S, Schneider N, et al: Determinants of deranged sodium and water homeostasis in decompensated cirrhosis. *J Lab Clin Med* 87:822–839, 1976
5. Berlyne G M, Sutton J, Brown C, et al: Renal salt and water handling in water immersion in the nephrotic syndrome. *Clin Sci* 61:605–610, 1981
6. Brown C, Sutton J V, Adler A J, et al: Renal calcium and magnesium handling in water immersion in nephrotic syndrome. *Nephron* 33:17–20, 1983
7. Berlyne G M, Sutton J V, Brown C, et al: Renal handling of urate during water immersion in the nephrotic syndrome. *Mineral Electrolyte Metab* 10:259–262, 1984

14

Treatment of Idiopathic Membranous Glomerulopathy

JEROME G. PORUSH AND PIERRE F. FAUBERT

> *"You cannot be sure of the success of your remedy while you are still uncertain of the nature of the disease."*
> Peter Mere Latham (1789–1875)

INTRODUCTION

The management of idiopathic membranous glomerulopathy (IMG) continues to be wrapped in controversy despite the fact that it is histologically one of the best defined glomerular diseases. This parodox was recently emphasized by Glassock[1] who proposed that the disease entity of IMG is very likely the common morphological expression of several diseases, which may have different responses to therapy, ostensibly related to different specific etiologies and pathogenetic processes. Until the specific etiology in each patient with IMG is recognized, it is likely that the therapy of this disease entity will remain essentially empirical.

The controversy with regard to corticosteroid therapy (and cytotoxic agents) has arisen from the conflicting results available, primarily from a literature containing mainly retrospective studies in which there are often a large variety of uncontrolled factors contributing to the results. This problem becomes particularly important in a disease such as membranous glomerulopathy in which some spontaneous remissions occur although in other patients the disease progressively worsens either rapidly or slowly and in still others remains stable for long periods of time.

In the present chapter we attempt to define the natural history of

JEROME G. PORUSH AND PIERRE F. FAUBERT • Division of Nephrology and Hypertension, The Brookdale Hospital Medical Center, Brooklyn, New York 11212.

IMG by analyzing untreated patients reported in the literature. By analyzing the results in treated patients (corticosteroids and/or cytotoxic agents), we attempt to answer the question whether these agents are indeed useful and develop a treatment strategy, if possible. In order to avoid some of the many pitfalls we have encountered in our review, we have concentrated on only those studies in which there are patients described with sufficient detail to permit us to take into account those factors that we believe may be responsible for some of the conflicting results, as outlined in Table I. In any particular series we have used primarily those patients who meet the criteria we have established below. We have restricted ourselves to studies published during the past 15 years in which the morphological diagnosis of membranous glomerulopathy has been rather precise. We have included the morphological stage wherever possible and have attempted to correlate this with outcome. We have included only patients with IMG and have excluded any patient in whom there was an underlying condition that might have been associated with membranous glomerulopathy, such as carcinoma, heavy metal exposure, etc. We have been able, in many instances, to exclude the complications described in Table I, item 8, which may account for progessive renal failure.

Finally, we used only those patients in whom the dose of prednisone or its equivalent could be determined with a fair degree of accuracy either by specific statement or indirectly by case histories. We used a total dose of 1800 mg (and at least 4 weeks of therapy) as the minimum dose necessary for inclusion. This dose level was used in fewer than 5% of patients, and most patients received much larger doses. We excluded patients under age 15 whenever possible, so that in this analysis the number of children (under age 15) is less than 5%. The male : female ra-

Table I. Factors Influencing the Outcome and Effects of Therapy in
Membranous Glomerulopathy

1. Precise morphological diagnosis and stage of disease
2. Heterogeneous patient mix: secondary forms and idiopathic variety must be distinguished
3. Better prognosis in children versus adults
4. Better prognosis in women versus men?
5. Duration of disease prior to diagnosis and length of follow-up
6. Clinical findings at entry
7. Outcome criteria used
8. Complications: renal vein thrombosis, interstitial nephritis secondary to diuretics, supervention of crescentic nephritis
9. Specific type, dosage, and duration of therapy

tio is shown in most instances, and follow-up time is relatively long, with the majority of patients followed for more than 4 years. Patients with short follow-up time were included when outcome was clearly evident, such as when patients had rapidly progressive renal failure or when it would have been necessary to exclude an entire series because of a small number of patients with a short follow-up.

For all patients utilized in this analysis, we had sufficient information with regard to proteinuria and renal function to be confident of their clinical status at entry and at final observation. In the study of Ehrenreich et al.[2] we were able to review the original raw data and greatly expand the information base beyond that given in the published paper. In this study, as in other series, outcome was often discussed in terms of proteinuria only so that a patient who had a significant decrease in proteinuria might be considered to have improved even though renal function concurrently deteriorated. In other studies, patients with persistent nephrotic syndrome with or without therapy were lumped together with patients who had progressive renal failure and were thereby considered to have a poor long-term prognosis. In the present analysis, these confusing issues were avoided by examining the outcome on last observation with specific reference to the degree of proteinuria and the level of renal function and treating these parameters separately.

In addition to taking into account the factors outlined in Table I, we felt that an additional factor that may have led to the conflicting results in retrospective studies was that patients with a variety of initial clinical findings were usually lumped together without regard to the possibility that prognosis and response to therapy might be related to these initial differences. Therefore, for the development of "historical" control groups and for the corticosteroid-treated patients, we carried out the analysis in three groups: (1) patients with nonnephrotic proteinuria and normal kidney function, (2) patients with nephrotic syndrome and preserved kidney function, and (3) patients with decreased renal function. For precise definitions of these groups, see Table II. This table also defines outcome criteria and provides the definition for decreased kidney function that we used for grouping patients on entry and as an outcome criterion. Any deviation from these definitions is noted.

With the above considerations in mind, we reviewed the literature and have included in the present analysis 12 retrospective studies[2-13] and six prospective studies,[14-19] all of which included treated and untreated patients except for Noel et al.[11] In some of these studies, either corticosteroids or cytotoxic agents were utilized, but in most corticosteroids and cytotoxic agents were used in various combinations in a proportion of patients.

Table II. Definitions

1. Nonnephrotic proteinuria: proteinuria <3.0–3.5 g/24 h
2. Nephrotic syndrome: proteinuria >3.0–3.5 g/24 h with or without hypoalbuminemia and edema
3. Normal or preserved renal function: serum creatinine ≤1.5 mg/dl and/or creatinine clearance ≥65 ml/min (unless stated otherwise)
4. Decreased renal function: serum creatinine >1.5 mg/dl and/or creatinine clearance <65 ml/min
5. Complete remission: proteinuria <0.2 g/24 h
6. Partial remission: proteinuria decreased by 50% or more or to 0.2–2.0 g/24 h with preserved renal function
7. Stable: no change in proteinuria or renal function

Table III summarizes the findings of Noel et al.[11] which we elected to describe separately because of the large number of untreated patients that could be adequately analyzed (116) and the relatively long follow-up period (54 months). The patients had a mean age of 38 years, and there were 52% males. We divided the patients into two groups. One contained 28 with nonnephrotic proteinuria, and the other had 88 patients with nephrotic syndrome. There were seven patients with moderate renal insufficency and seven who were 15 years old or less who could not be individually identified and may be in either subgroup. It is apparent that the 28 patients with nonnephrotic proteinuria did only slightly better than

Table III. Clinical Findings, Morphological Stage, and Outcome in 116 Untreated Adult Patients with Idiopathic Membranous Glomerulopathy[a]

	88 nephrotic syndrome	28 nonnephrotic proteinuria
Total patients (n)	116	
Mean age[b] (years)	38	
Males (%)	52	
Follow-up (months)	54 (2–252)	
Clinical status[c]	88 nephrotic syndrome	28 nonnephrotic proteinuria
Morphological stage		
I	15 (17%)	7 (25%)
II	64 (73%)	15 (54%)
III	9 (10%)	6 (21%)
Outcome		
Complete remission	21 (24%)	6 (21%)
Partial remission	10 (11%)	7 (25%)
Stable	37 (42%)	13 (47%)
Renal failure[d]	20 (23%)	2 (7%)

[a]Noel et al.,[11]
[b]Seven were 15 years old or less.
[c]Seven (all adults) had moderate renal insufficiency at time of biopsy.
[d]Eleven (50%) reached end-stage renal failure.

the 88 nephrotic patients with regard to achieving a complete or partial remission (46% versus 35%), whereas there were three times as many who developed progressive renal failure in the nephrotic group (23% versus 7%). Of the 22 patients with renal failure at outcome, seven had moderate renal insufficiency when first seen . Eleven of the 22 renal failure patients reached end-stage renal disease. In the 15 patients who had normal kidney function to start, renal failure developed fairly rapidly (mean 2.1 years), with only one patient developing renal insufficiency after 5 years of observation.

NONNEPHROTIC PROTEINURIA

Table IV summarizes our analysis of patients from retrospective studies who met the criteria we established of nonnephrotic proteinuria with normal or preserved renal function. Thirty-nine untreated patients from eight studies[2,3,5-9,13] and 22 corticosteroid-treated patients from five studies[2,5,6,9,13] were identified. The minimum total dose was 2500 mg of prednisone or equivalent, with most patients receiving a much higher dose (4–5 times). The mean age was similar in the two groups, and they were both followed for more than 7 years, with the treated group having a larger number of males (68% versus 59%). At the time of last observation, there was a similar percentage of complete remissions (38 and 41). In the treated group, a smaller percentage remained stable (27 versus

Table IV. Clinical Findings and Outcome in Adult Patients with Idiopathic Membranous Glomerulopathy with Nonnephrotic Proteinuria Only[a]: Retrospective Studies

	Untreated[b]	Steroid treated[c]
Number	39	22
Mean age (years)	37 ($n = 16$)	36 ($n = 19$)
Males (%)	59 ($n = 16$)	68 ($n = 19$)
Follow-up (months)	85	96
Outcome		
Complete remission	15 (38%)	9 (41%)
Stable	17 (44%)	6 (27%)
NS and/or RF[d]	7 (18%)	7 (32%)

[a]Proteinuria <3.0–3.5 g/24 h with normal or preserved renal function.
[b]From Pollack et al.,[3] Erwin et al.,[5] Franklin et al.,[6] Gluck et al.,[7] Row et al.,[8] Ehrenreich et al.,[2] Pierides et al.,[9] and Hopper et al.[13]
[c]From Erwin et al.,[5] Franklin et al.,[6] Ehrenreich et al.,[2] Pierides et al.,[9] and Hopper et al.[13] Prednisone dose 30–100 mg/24 h for 2 months or longer (up to 36 months); minimum total dose 2500 mg.
[d]NS, nephrotic syndrome; RF, renal failure.

44), and a higher percentage developed nephrotic syndrome and/or renal failure (32 versus 18). Because of the small number of patients, it would not seem reasonable to suggest that the corticosteroid-treated patients actually did worse.

Table V summarizes the data from the only prospective study of nonnephrotic proteinuria in which nine patients were untreated with a follow-up of 24 ± 17 months and nine patients were treated with prednisone and followed for 42 ± 17 months. This was not a randomized study but rather a sequential one in which nine patients were treated and then a subsequent group of nine were not treated. Prednisone therapy consisted of 30 mg per day for 2 months initially and then gradually tapered over 2 years with the same regimen used in each of the treated patients (25 mg/day for 2 months, 20 mg/day for 2 months, 15 mg/day for 6 months, 20 mg every other day for 6 months, and 15 mg every other day for 6 months). The age of the untreated patients was 42 ± 12 compared to 36 ± 7 years in the treated group. There were 67% males in the

Table V. Clinical findings, Morphological Stage, and Outcome
in Adult Patients with Idiopathic Membranous Glomerulopathy With
Nonnephrotic Proteinuria Only[a] (Prospective Study)[b]

	Untreated	Steroid treated[c]
Number	9	9
Age (years)	42 ± 12(SD)	36 ± 7
Males (%)	67	22
Initial creatinine clearance (ml/min)	96 ± 11	104 ± 12
Initial proteinuria (g/24 h)	0.7 ± 0.6	0.8 ± 0.6
Morphological stage		
I	2	2
II	2	2
III	4	4
IV	1	1
Follow-up (months)		
Before entry	17 ± 22	17 ± 19
After entry	24 ± 19	42 ± 17
Outcome		
Final creatinine clearance (ml/min)	94 ± 8	104 ± 14
Final proteinuria (g/24 h)	1.1 ± 0.8 one transient complete remission)	six complete remissions and three unchanged, two of whom had transient complete remissions

[a]Proteinuria <3.5 g/24 h with normal renal function (creatinine clearance 82–122 ml/min).
[b]Kobayashi et al.[18]
[c]Prednisone 30 mg/day for 2 months and gradually tapered over 2 years.

untreated but only 22% in the treated group. The initial creatinine clearance and degree of proteinuria were similar in the two groups, as was the morphological staging by electron microscopy. At final observation, both groups had similar creatinine clearances. In the untreated group, proteinuria was similar to the initial level (1.1 ± 0.8 versus 0.7 ± 0.6 g/24 h), and only one of the nine patients had a transient complete remission; however, in the treated group, six patients had a complete remission, and two of the other three had transient complete remissions.

Thus, the treated patients in this study appeared to do better than the untreated patients in this study as well as the untreated patients with nonnephrotic proteinuria described by Noel et al.[11] (Table III) and the untreated and treated patients analyzed from other retrospective studies (Table IV). It should be noted, however, that this is a rather small series, and seven of the nine (78%) of the treated patients were female compared to 59% males in the retrospective series and probably about 50% in the Noel series (exact percentage of males in the nonnephrotic proteinuric group not clearly defined, but there were 52% in the entire series). If it is true that females do better than males, as suggested by Hopper et al,[13] this might explain the excellent results in the treated patients in the Kobayashi study. Most studies, however, do not show a more benign course in females or suggest that they respond to therapy better.

NEPHROTIC PROTEINURIA

The bulk of the patients seen in most of the published series of membranous nephropathy present with nephrotic syndrome with preserved or normal renal function (as defined above). Table VI summarizes our analysis of untreated patients from seven retrospective studies[2,4-6,8,9,13] in which we were able to identify 91 patients with nephrotic syndrome and preserved renal function. It is likely that there were a few patients included in this analysis with mild renal insufficiency (probably no more than 5%) and a few (3–5) patients who were under age 15 who could not be excluded without excluding the entire study. These patients had a mean age of 44 ($n = 59$), and there were 64% males ($n = 59$). The mean follow-up was 70 months, with the shortest series (four patients) followed 33 months and the longest series (16 patients) followed 99 months. In this group of 91 patients with nephrotic syndrome, 36% had complete or partial remission, 22% remained stable, and 42% developed renal failure. The results of this analysis are quite similar to those of Noel et al.[11] (Table III) with regard to the percentage of patients with nephrotic syndrome who had a complete or partial remission; however, the patients

Table VI. Clinical Findings and Outcome in Untreated Adult Patients with Idiopathic Membranous Glomerulopathy and Nephrotic Syndrome with Preserved Renal Function[a]: Retrospective Studies

Author	Number	Males (%)	Mean age (years)	Follow-up (months)	Outcome		
					CR or PR[b]	S[c]	↓RF[d]
Hayslett	7	71	34	57	1	4	2
Erwin	17	71	49	60	4	6	7
Franklin	4	50	45	33	—	—	4
Row	20	NA[e]	NA	75	5	1	14
Ehrenreich	16	56	44	99	11	4	1
Pierides	12	NA	NA	60	5	4	3
Hopper	15	60	44	71	7	1	7
Total	91	64 ($n=59$)	44 ($n=59$)	70	33 (36%)	20 (22%)	38 (42%)

[a]Serum creatinine ≤1.5 mg/dl and/or creatinine clearance ≥65 ml/min.
[b]CR, complete remission; PR, partial remission.
[c]S, stable.
[d]↓RF, decreased renal function.
[e]NA, not available.

included in this analysis did somewhat worse with regard to renal function. Forty-two percent of patients developed renal failure, which is more in keeping with the generally held view that approximately 50% of patients with membranous glomerulopathy will progress to renal failure either fairly rapidly (within 5 years of onset) or more slowly (5–15 years or longer after onset).

Table VII summarizes our analysis of 162 patients with nephrotic syndrome and preserved renal function, identified from ten retrospective studies,[2,4,-10,12,13] who received prednisone or its equivalent with a minimum total dose of 1800 mg (in only a few patients). The majority of patients received four or more times this amount. The mean age of the patients was 40 years ($n = 129$) with 58% males ($n = 129$), both similar to the untreated patients described above. The mean follow-up was 79 months ($n = 141$), with the shortest series (20 patients) followed 48 months and the longest (six patients) followed 128 months. Ninety-two patients (57%) had a complete remission, and only 46 (28%) developed renal failure, with 24 (15%) remaining stable. These results contrast favorably with the analysis of 91 untreated patients described in Table VI. In general, patients tolerated corticosteroids very well even for long periods of time.

In 1970, Black, Rose, and Brewer[20] reported the results of a prospective randomized controlled trial of prednisone in 195 adult patients with nephrotic syndrome, of whom 19 were classified as membranous glomerulopathy. Unfortunately, because of the inability to identify individual patients precisely, the lack of precise status at entry (proteinuria versus nephrotic syndrome with or without renal failure), the relatively small daily dose of prednisone (20–30 mg/day, although for up to 6 months), and difficulties with establishing a precise morphological diagnosis in all cases (a relative large number of discrepancies between two pathologists), these patients cannot be used for the present analysis.

Table VIII summarizes the results from the United States Collaborative Study of Adult Idiopathic Nephrotic Syndrome published in 1979.[17] Up to that time there were 72 patients with IMG, of whom 38 were randomly assigned to the placebo group and 34 to the steroid-treated group in a double-blind study. Nephrotic syndrome was defined as ≥ 3.5g/24 h per 1.73 m^2 of proteinuria, and "normal" renal function as a creatinine clearance of ≥ 60 liters/24 h (42 ml/min), which is much lower than most other studies as well as being lower than the criteria established for our retrospective series of nephrotic syndrome described in Tables VI and VII. Most of the patients had a serum creatinine under 1.5 mg/dl with 1.0 ± 0.2 in the placebo group and 1.1 ± 0.2 mg/dl in the corticosteroid treated group. Corticosteroid therapy consisted of 100–150 mg of prednisone every other day (125 mg for patients weighing 45–80 kg)

Table VII. Clinical Findings and Outcome in Steroid-Treated[a] Adult Patients with Idiopathic Membranous Glomerulopathy and Nephrotic Syndrome with Preserved Renal Function[b]: Retrospective Studes

Author	Number	Males (%)	Mean age (years)	Follow-up (months)	Outcome		
					CR or PR[c]	S[d]	↓RF[e]
Hayslett	7	43	29	51	2	3	2
Erwin	18	72	48	53	7	6	5
Franklin	15	73	38	73	3	—	12
Gluck	16	NA[f]	NA	NA	3	5	8
Row	6	NA	NA	61	1	2	3
Ehrenreich	28	54	38	76	21	3	4
Pierides	6	NA	NA	128	4	—	2
Bolton	20	70	39	48	15	5	—
Suki	5	NA	NA	NA	5	—	—
Hopper	41	46	40	112	31	—	10
Total	162	58 (n = 129)	40 (n = 129)	79(n = 141)	92 (57%)	24 (15%)	46 (28%)

[a] Prednisone dose 30–100 mg/day for 6 weeks or longer (up to 36 months); minimum total dose 1800 mg.
[b] Serum creatinine ≤1.5 mg/dl and/or creatinine clearance ≥65 ml/min.
[c] CR, complete remission; PR, partial remission.
[d] S, stable.
[e] ↓RF, decreased renal function.
[f] NA, not available.

Table VIII. Clinical Findings, Morphological Stage, and Outcome in Adult Patients with Idiopathic Membranous Glomerulopathy with Nephrotic Syndrome[a] and Relatively Good Kidney Function[b,c]

	Placebo	Steroid treated[d]
Number	38	34
Mean age (years)		
16–30	15	9
31–45	10	14
46–65	13	11
Males (%)	53	65
Admission serum creatinine (mg/dl)	1.0 ± 0.2(SD)	1.1 ± 0.2
Admission proteinuria (g/24 h)	8.3 ± 4	9.4 ± 6
Morphological stage		
I	9	5
II	20	18
III–IV	8	9
Intermediate	1	2
Follow-up (months)	23	23
Outcome		
ΔGFR	– 10%/year	– 2%/year $(P < 0.02)$
Creatinine stop point[e]	11 (29%)	2 (6%) $(P = 0.01)$
Proteinuria remission rate		
(complete or partial)[f]	11 (29%)	22 (65%) $(P < 0.01)$

[a]Defined as ≥ 3.5 g/24 h per 1.73 m^2 of proteinuria.
[b]Defined as a creatinine clearance ≥ 60 liters/24 h (42 ml/min) per 1.73 m^2.
[c]Collaborative Study.[17]
[d]Prednisone 100–150 mg every other day (125 mg for 45–80 kg body weight) for 2 months and tapered over 1 month if no remission and over 2 months if a remission was noted.
[e]Doubling of serum creatinine (two measurements). In the placebo group all 11 progressed, whereas in the steroid-treated group one of two went on to dialysis, and one stabilized with a serum creatinine of 2.3 mg/dl.
[f]Most of the remissions were transient, so that there was no difference between groups at "final" observation.

for 2 months and tapered over one additional month if there was no remission (complete or partial) and tapered over 2 months if a remission was noted. Patients were retreated if a relapse occurred after a partial or complete remission. The mean age of the patients was similar, but the placebo group had somewhat more patients under age 30. The degree of proteinuria was similar, 8.3 ± 4 and 9.4 ± 6 g/24 h in the placebo and treated groups, respectively, as was the morphological staging, with the majority of patients in stage II in both groups. The follow-up time was relatively short, with a mean of 23 months and the longest only 52 months.

Nevertheless, there was a clear-cut difference in the groups. The creatinine clearance (GFR) decreased at a higher rate in the placebo group, – 10%/year compared to – 2%/year in the treated group

($P < 0.02$). Eleven of 38 (29%) reached a creatinine "stop point" in the former (defined as a doubling of serum creatinine, two measurements), whereas only two of 34 (6%) reached a creatinine "stop point" in the steroid treated group ($P = 0.01$). In the placebo group, in all 11 patients renal function progressively deteriorated after the creatinine "stop point" was reached, whereas in the treated group, one of the two went on to dialysis, and one stabilized with a serum creatinine of 2.3 mg/dl. Finally, a significantly larger number of patients in the treated group had a partial or complete remission, 22 of 34 (65%) compared to only 11 of 38 (29%) in the placebo group ($P < 0.01$); however, at the time of last observation, the number of patients in remission in the treated group was not significantly greater than in the placebo group. On longer follow-up (60 months), the treated patients have continued to do well, and the number who have had a partial or complete remission is now significantly greater than the placebo group (C.H. Coggins, personal communication). In general, the treatment was very well tolerated with minimal side effects.

Cattran et al.[19] in a preliminary report of a prospective controlled study of 79 adults with IMG, using approximately 80 mg/1.7 m^2 of prednisone every other day for 6 months (32 treated, 47 control), noted that patients with stage I or II benefited from therapy in terms of preservation of GFR, with no significant difference between treated and control stage III–IV patients. There was no significant difference in proteinuria between groups. As in the initial report of the United States Collaborative Study, the follow-up period was relatively short, averaging less than 2 years. There were minimal side effects of therapy even though the total dose of prednisone was approximately 7 g, almost twice the total dose utilized in the United States Collaborative Study.

RENAL FAILURE

Table IX summarizes the findings in patients with IMG with renal failure, as defined above. We included patients with or without nephrotic amounts of proteinuria. In this analysis, we found 25 untreated patients in five retrospective studies[2,4-6,13] and 32 treated patients in four retrospective studies.[2,5,10,13] Unfortunately, there are no published results of a prospective controlled study in IMG patients with renal failure. There were no differences in mean age between the groups or percentage of males, which was relatively high, 72% and 78% in the untreated and treated groups, respectively. The follow-up period was 54 months in the untreated and 78 months in the treated. The striking finding was that none of the untreated patients had a remission of proteinuria and 23 (92%) had progressive renal failure, with only two pa-

Table IX. Clinical Findings and Outcome in Adult Patients with Idiopathic Membranous Glomerulopathy and Renal Failure[a]: Retrospective Studies

	Untreated[b]	Steroid treated[c]
Number	25	32
Mean age (years)	54	48 ($n = 28$)
Males (%)	72	78 ($n = 28$)
Mean serum creatinine (mg/dl)	5.5	2.5
Follow-up (months)	54	87 ($n = 28$)
Outcome		
Remission, complete or partial, and/or improved renal function	—	17 (53%)
Stable	2 (8%)	3 (9%)
Progressive renal failure	23 (92%)	12 (38%)

[a]Serum creatinine ≥ 1.5 mg/dl and/or creatinine clearance ≤ 65 ml/min.
[b]From Hayslett et al.,[4] Erwin et al.,[5] Franklin et al.,[6] Ehrenreich et al.,[2] and Hopper et al.[13]
[c]From Erwin et al.,[5] Ehrenreich et al.,[2] Bolton et al.,[10] and Hopper et al.[13] Prednisone dose 30–100 mg/day for 6 weeks or longer (up to several years); minimum total dose 2500 mg.

tients remaining stable. In the treated group, 17 (53%) had a complete or partial remission and/or improved renal function, with 12 (38%) becoming progressively worse and three (9%) remaining stable. The only factor that makes interpretation of these findings precarious was that the untreated patients had a much higher mean serum creatinine, 5.5 compared to 2.5 mg/dl in the treated group. There was overlap between groups, however, and within the treated group, there was no correlation between the level of serum creatinine and response to therapy.

CYTOTOXIC DRUGS

The final group examined were patients treated with cytotoxic agents with or without prednisone. In five retrospective studies,[2,4,8,9,12] summarized in Table X, 48 patients were included, of whom 41 received prednisone and cyclophosphamide and/or azathioprine and seven received cyclophosphamide alone (six from Pierides et al.[9] and one from Ehrenreich et al.[2]). In general, patients received prednisone prior to or in conjunction with cyclophosphamide or azathioprine. It would appear that in a few instances prednisone may have been continued after the cytotoxic agent was discontinued. Most of the patients had nephrotic syndrome, and only four patients (8%) had mild to moderate renal failure (serum creatinine 1.6–30 mg/dl). The mean age was 36 ($n = 18$), and 50% were males ($n = 18$). They were followed for 71 months ($n = 34$). Thirty-three patients (69%) had a complete or partial remission, three of whom received cyclophosphamide alone, and 15 (31%) had no remission or worsening renal function, with most in the latter category. These pa-

Table X. Clinical Findings and Outcome in Adult Patients with Idiopathic Membranous Glomerulopathy Treated with Cytotoxic Agents with or without Prednisone[a]: Retrospective Studies

Author	Therapy[b]	Number	Mean age (years)	Males (%)	Follow-up (months)	Outcome	
						CR or PR[c]	NR[d]
Hayslett	PA	6	41	50	57	5	1
Row	PA,PC,PAC	8	NA[e]	NA	77	4	4
Ehrenreich	PA,PC,C	12	33	50	67	9	3
Pierides	PAC,C	8	NA	NA	83	4	4
Suki	PA,PC	14	NA	NA	NA	11	3
Total		48	36 ($n=18$)	50 ($n=18$)	71 ($n=34$)	33 (69%)	15 (31%)

[a]Only 8% had a decrease in renal function (serum creatinine 1.6–3.0 mg/dl) initially.
[b]P, prednisone; C, cyclophosphamide; A, azathioprine. Dose of P 30–60 mg/day for 3 months or longer; dose of A or C 1.5–3.0 mg/kg per day for at least 6 months.
[c]CR, complete remission; PR, partial remission.
[d]NR, no remission and/or worsening renal function.
[e]NA, not available.

tients did much better than the untreated patients with nephrotic syndrome described by Noel et al.[11] (Table III) and the untreated patients with nephrotic syndrome in the retrospective studies (Table VI). They also appeared to do slightly better than the corticosteroid-treated nephrotic patients in the retrospective studies (Table VII).

Table XI summarizes the experience in three prospective studies[14-16] in which a cytotoxic agent was used alone and compared to an untreated control group. In the study by Donadio et al.[14] most of the patients had nephrotic syndrome with preserved renal function, with two patients in each group having proteinuria only and an unspecified number with a decrease in renal function (highest serum creatinine 2.2 mg/dl and lowest creatinine clearance 33 ml/min). Some of the patients had received corticosteroid therapy, but none for a 30-day period prior to admission into the study. After 1 year of therapy, consisting of cyclophosphamide 1.5–2.5 mg/kg per day, the GFR was stable in both groups with no significant difference in remission rate between the two groups. Eight treated patients and seven untreated patients were followed for an additional 12 months with no significant change in clinical status in either group. The use of corticosteroids in some of the patients (unspecified as to number and group) makes interpretation of these data difficult.

In the study by Lagrue et al.[15] all of the patients had nephrotic syndrome and preserved renal function. Eleven patients received azathioprine, 3 mg/kg per day for 6 months followed by 2 mg/kg per day for 6 months; 16 patients received chlorambucil, 2 mg/kg per day for 6 months followed by 1 mg/kg per day for 6 months, and were compared

Table XI. Clinical Findings and Outcome in Adult Patients with Idiopathic Membranous Glomerulopathy Treated with Cytotoxic Agents: Prospective Studies

Author	Therapy[a]	Number	Mean age (years)	Males (%)	Follow-up (months)	Outcome CR or PR[b]	NR[c]
Donadio	C	11	43	82	12	3	8
	U	11	46	73	12	2	9
Lagrue	A	11	NA[d]	NA	12	1	10
	Cl	16	NA	NA	12	13	3
	U	14	NA	NA	12	3	11
Canadian	A	5	41	60	12	2	3
	U	4	45	75	12	1	3

[a]C, cyclophosphamide; A, azathioprine; Cl, chlorambucil; U, untreated controls.
[b]CR, complete remission; PR, partial remission.
[c]NR, no remission and/or worsening renal function.

to 14 untreated patients. After 1 year there was no difference between the azathioprine group and the control group; however, the patients who received chlorambucil did significantly better than the untreated controls, with 13 of 16 having a partial or complete remission compared to only three of the 14 control patients.

The final prospective study by the Western Canadian Glomerulonephritis Study Group[16] also employed azathioprine, 2.5 mg/kg per day for 12 months in five patients and compared the outcome at 1 year with four placebo-treated patients. All patients had >3 g/24 proteinuria and a creatinine clearance >50 ml/min. Two of the five treated patients had a partial or complete remission and, as a group, had a significant decrease in proteinuria, whereas only one of the four untreated patients had a partial remission without worsening renal function, and, as a group, the BUN increased significantly. As in the Donadio study, some of the patients had previously received corticosteroids, but none for at least 4 months prior to the study. In general, in this study as well as the other two prospective studies, there were relatively few side effects attributed to the cytotoxic drugs.

MORPHOLOGICAL STAGING

The correlation between morphological stage and outcome in treated and untreated patients is summarized in Table XII. Included are only those studies in which sufficient data are given to compare morphological stage at entry with outcome in treated and/or untreated patients. In almost all the studies staging was according to the criteria established by Ehrenreich and Churg[21] with or without minor variations. In general, there was no clear-cut correlation between the pathological stage on entry and outcome; however, there was a tendency for stage I and II patients to do better than patients with more advanced lesions, whether treated or not. It should be noted that most of the patients examined in all of the studies had either stage I or II lesions, so that there was not a sufficiently large number of patients with advanced lesions to allow confidence about the true significance of this finding.

TREATMENT STRATEGIES

The primary object of the analyses carried out was to develop a strategy for the treatment of adult IMG. The results of the present detailed analysis are far from clear-cut because of the continued depen-

Table XII. Correlation between Morphological Stage and Outcome in Treatd and Nontreated Patients

Retrospective studies	
Hayslett	No correlation.
Erwin	No overall correlation; patients with earlier lesion tended to do better.
Franklin	No correlation with EM staging; however, all six remissions occurred in patients with 1–2 + BM thickening on light microscopy, and those who did poorly generally had 3–4 + BM thickening.
Gluck	No overall correlation, but remissions seen only in stage I or II patients.
Row	No correlation.
Ehrenreich	Greater percentage of stage I and II went into remission than stage III. No remission in stage IV patients.
Pierides	No correlation.
Noel	Using light microscopy primarily with classifications adopted from Bariety et al.,[22] types I and II had more remissions than type III patients. No ESRD in type I.
Cattran	Stage I and II treated patients did better than stage I and II untreated patients in terms of preservation of GFR. No difference between treated and untreated in stage III and IV.
Prospective studies	
U.S. Collaborative Study	No correlation.
Kobayashi	No correlation.
Donadio	No correlation.

dence on retrospective studies (to some degree) and also the lack of information with regard to specific etiologies and incomplete understanding of pathogenic events. Nevertheless, there would appear to be sufficient data from both the present retrospective analysis and the prospective controlled studies to develop a strategy for treatment. Since we considered it important to define the specific clinical status of patients on entry in an attempt to circumvent some of the confusion in the literature, we are able to discuss treatment strategies in defined groups.

In nonnephrotic proteinuria, no therapy is recommended unless the patient progresses to nephrotic proteinuria or develops renal failure (see below).

In nephrotic syndrome with preserved renal function, a course of prednisone of 125 mg every other day if the patient weighs 45–80 kg (150 mg for more than 80 kg and 100 mg for less than 45 kg) for 2 months with tapering on a weekly or biweekly basis for two additional months would appear to be a reasonable approach. If the patient has a remission and exacerbates, retreatment is recommended. If the patient persists with troublesome nephrotic syndrome after the 2 months of full therapy, a longer course of prednisone should be undertaken. The treatment may be continued for a year or longer depending on the patient's tolerance. The dose should be tapered gradually over this period of time (taking into consideration side effects and clinical response). This approach is similar to that suggested by Glassock[1] for patients in this category. If the patient is prednisone resistant and still has troublesome nephrotic syndrome, cyclosphosphamide or azathioprine may be added. It is not possible to sort out with any precision how these drugs were combined or exactly what dose of prednisone to recommend after the patient is placed on the cytotoxic agent. Generally, the dose of prednisone was lower than the initial dose, of the order of 20–40 mg per day, when given in conjunction with cyclophosphamide or azathioprine.

For decreased renal function, the results of the present analysis in this category of IMG provide some interesting data not previously available, which permit us to recommend a treatment strategy. If the renal failure is mild to moderate (perhaps up to a serum creatinine of 4 to 5 mg/dl), an initial course of prednisone as described in the previous group would seem reasonable. If well tolerated, prednisone may be continued for a longer period of time with tapering of the dose dependent on the response. There are insufficient data to base an opinion with regard to the use of cytotoxic agents in combination with a corticosteroid in this category of IMG if there is no improvement with corticosteroid therapy alone. This is an area deserving of further testing, which, in fact, is being done by the United States Collaborative Study Group.

At the present time there are no data suggesting a role for cyclophosphamide or azathioprine alone in patients with nephrotic syndrome with or without renal failure. Chlorambucil, however, deserves further testing.

ACKNOWLEDGMENT. We wish to acknowledge the invaluable secretarial assistance of Pauline Kleiman, Pauline Wernick, and Ruth Porush.

REFERENCES

1. Glassock RJ: Corticosteroid therapy is beneficial in adults with idiopathic membranous glomerulopathy. Am J Kidney Dis 1:376–385, 1982
2. Ehrenreich T, Porush JG, Churg J, et al: Treatment of idiopathic membranous nephropathy. N Engl J Med 295:741–746, 1976
3. Pollack VE, Rosen S, Pirani CL, et al: Natural history of lipoid nephrosis and membranous glomerulonephritis. Ann Inter Med 67:1171–1191, 1968
4. Hayslett FP, Kashgarian M, Bensch KG, et al: Clinicopathologic correlations in nephrotic syndrome due to primary renal disease. Medicine 52:93–120, 1973

5. Erwin DT, Donadio JV, Holley KE: The clinical course of idiopathic membranous nephropathy. *Mayo Clin Proc* 48:697-712, 1973
6. Franklin WA, Jennings RB, Earle DP: Membranous glomerulopenritis: Long-term serial observations on clinical course and morphology. *Kidney Int* 4:36-56, 1973
7. Gluck MC, Gallo G, Lowenstein J, et al: Membranous glomerulonephritis. Evolution of clinical and pathologic features. *Ann Intern Med* 78:1-12, 1973
8. Row RG, Cameron JS, Turner DR, et al: Membranous nephropathy. Long term followup and association with neoplasia. *Q J Med* 44(174):207-239, 1975
9. Pierides AM, Malasit P, Morley AR, et al: Idiopathic membranous nephropathy. *Q J Med* 46(182):163-177, 1977
10. Bolton WK, Atuk NO, Sturgill BC, et al: Therapy of the idiopathic nephrotic syndrome (INS) with alternate day steroids. *Am J Med* 62:60-70, 1977
11. Noel LH, Zanetti M, Droz D, et al: Long term prognosis of idiopathic membranous glomerulonephritis. Study of 116 untreated patients. *Am J Med* 66:82-90, 1979
12. Suki WN, Chavez A: Membraneous nephropathy: Response to steroids and immunosuppression. *Am J Nephrol* 1:11-16, 1981
13. Hopper J Jr, Trew PA, Biava CG: Membranous nephropathy: Its relative benignity in women. *Nephron* 29:18-24, 1981
14. Donadio JV Jr, Holley KE, Anderson CF, et al: Controlled trial of cyclophosphamide in idiopathic membranous nephropathy. *Kidney Int* 6:431-439, 1974
15. Lagrue G, Bernard D, Bariety J, et al: Traitment par le chlorambucil et l'azathioprine dan les glomerulonephrites primitives. *J Urol Nephrol* 9:655-672, 1975
16. Western Canadian Glomerulonephritis Study Group: Controlled trial of azathiaprine in the nephrotic syndrome secondary to idiopathic membranous glomerulonephritis. *Can Med Assoc J* 115:1209-1210, 1976
17. Collaborative Study of the Adult Idiopathic Nephrotic Syndrome: A controlled study of short term prednisone treatment in adults with membranous nephropathy. *N Engl J Med* 301:1301-1306, 1979
18. Kobayashi Y, Tateno S, Shigematsu H, et al: Prednisone treatment in non nephrotic patients with idiopathic membranous nephropathy. *Nephron* 30:210-219, 1982
19. Cattran D, Cardella C, Charron R, et al: Preliminary results of controlled trial of alternate day prednisone (ADS) in idiopathic membranous glomerulonephritis (IMGN). Presented at 8th International Congress of Nephrology, Athens, June 7-12, 1981, Abstract CN-146
20. Black DAK, Rose G, Brewer DB: Controlled trial of prednisone in adult patients with the nephrotic syndrome. *Br Med J* 3:421-426, 1970
21. Ehrenreich T, Churg J: Pathology of membranous nephropathy. *Pathol Ann* 3:145-186, 1968
22. Bariety J, Druet P, Lagrue G, et al: Les glomérulonéphrites "extramembraneuses" (GEM): Étude morphologique en microscopic optique, électronique et immunofluorescence. *Pathol Biol* 18:5-32, 1970

15

Malignant Proteinuria
A Newly Described Syndrome and Its Management with Medical Nephrectomy

M. M. AVRAM

INTRODUCTION

From our own cases and cases reported by others emerges our clinical recognition that a new syndrome exists in patients with advanced uremia consisting of massive protein loss (over 25 g/day), to which we now give, for the first time, the designation "malignant proteinuria." It is a life-threatening syndrome.

The common final pathway of malignant proteinuria may result from a wide variety of histopathological and functional alterations ranging from focal sclerosis, as described in separate chapters in this book by J. E. Kiley and associates and others[1] reported elsewhere, by amyloid kidney following longstanding tuberculosis,[2] by excess renin,[3] and by glomerulopathy in the uremic[4] and the nonuremic transplanted kidney[5] (reportedly up to 120 g albumin in the urine collected in 24 h).

It is apparent that although focal sclerosis is the most frequent cause of malignant proteinuria, this massive protein loss can be encountered with minimal histological changes (mild increase in mesangial matrix) as well as with total glomerular destruction.

A multitude of other workers have, separately, dealt with this same group of patients or patients with tumors, recurrent urinary infections, or severe hypertension, utilizing various therapeutic regimens in its management. These regimens include bilateral nephrectomy, unilateral nephrectomy, embolization of renal artery with gel shreds, renal artery

M. M. AVRAM • Division of Nephrology, The Avram Center for Kidney Diseases, The Long Island College Hospital, Brooklyn, New York 11201; and Department of Medicine, State University of New York, Downstate Medical Center, Brooklyn, New York 11203.

occlusion with stainless steel, Swann–Ganz balloon occlusion, etc. All of these extraordinary measures were triggered by the presence in these very ill patients of malignant proteinuria (25 g protein/24 h or more). This massive proteinuria leads to markedly decreased serum albumin, causing, in turn, decreased plasma oncotic pressure, loss of fluid into the extravascular space, severely reduced plasma volume, and life-threatening hypotension and shock (see Fig. 1). If uncontrolled, this will lead to death. This lethal chain of events can be reversed in most cases only by the destruction of remnant nephrons, thus obliterating the source of malignant protein leakage in leaking glomeruli and in tubules no longer able to reabsorb any proteins.

The purpose of this chapter is twofold: to describe the existence of the "malignant proteinuria" syndrome and to review its management with a now confirmed modality of treatment, namely, medical nephrectomy using metallic salts.

In treating patients with chronic renal failure, the nephrologist usually attempts to preserve residual renal function as long as possible. However, there are certain situations in which the presence of the diseased kidneys becomes hazardous to the patient's well-being. Extirpation of the kidneys is often necessary in uremic patients with such complications as massive proteinuria,[1] malignant hypertension,[6-9] and recurrent urinary tract infection and hypertension.[10]

To treat desperately ill patients suffering with this deadly syndrome, desperate measures to reverse the massive proteinuria have been used, including gel foam embolization,[1] renal ablation with stainless steel coils,[11] aberrant uninephrectomy,[4] and even bilateral surgical nephrectomy.[7]

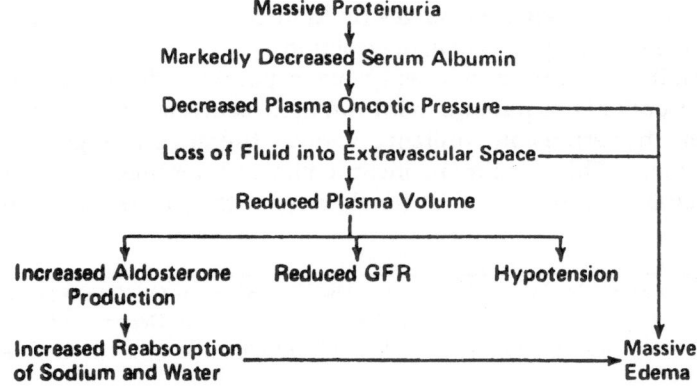

Figure 1. Physiological effects of malignant proteinuria.

As an alternative to surgery, we have developed a method of "medical nephrectomy" using a nephrotoxic agent to abolish kidney function.[2] We have had successful experience with this mode of therapy in uremic patients with massive proteinuria. Since our initial report, several personal communications and also more formal reports have confirmed our experience with the successful use of medical nephrectomy by other centers in the United States (J.E. Kiley et al., Chapter 16, this volume) and in other countries.

PATIENTS AND METHODS

Two patients were seen; each presented with massive proteinuria, hypoalbuminemia, severe hypotension, and, at times, shock. In order to reduce further life-threatening urinary protein loss, the mercurial salt mercaptomerin sodium was used with satisfactory results. A description of events leading to malignant proteinuria and medical nephrectomy follows:

Case No. 1. A 69-year-old male with a past history of tuberculosis 30 years prior to admission, while in a European concentration camp, was referred with uremia, anasarca, and hypotension. Laboratory tests revealed serum creatinine 14 mg/dl, serum albumin 1.4 g/dl, creatinine clearance 3 ml/min, and urinary protein 31 g/day. There was no longer any evidence of active tuberculosis. An immunoelectrophoresis was normal, with no paraproteins present. Quantitative immunoglobulins revealed a low normal IgG with normal IgA, IgM, and IgD. The serum protein electrophoresis revealed no abnormal spikes. The serum and urinary electrophoretic patterns were quite similar, suggesting low selectivity (Fig. 2). Serum complement level was normal. Bence Jones proteins were absent, and ANA and LE preps were negative. The bone marrow was normal, with no increase in plasma cells.

A renal biopsy revealed widespread amyloidosis in the glomeruli and blood vessels. Light microscopy showed large masses of amyloid replacing glomerular lobules (Fig. 3). The basement membranes of glomerular tufts outlined the lobules. A crystal violet stain of the same specimen showed metachromatic masses of amyloid replacing lobules. An electron micrograph showed the fine fibrillar structure of amyloid in the capillary tuft, obliterating the lumen (Figs. 4,5). Immunofluorescence revealed autofluorescent, pale green masses of amyloid within lobules but showed no specific staining for polyvalent γ-globulins. An earlier biopsy had shown amyloid (Fig. 6).

The patient was maintained on peritoneal dialysis, and an A–V fistula was created. Treatment was made difficult by the occurrence of hypotensive shock with minimal fluid removal and repeated clotting of the fistula. There was poor healing of the incision site because of local edema. The patient was given anabolic agents, a high-protein, essential amino acid diet, and a total of 500 g of salt-poor albumin, without significant improvement. Bilateral nephrectomy was counseled, but the patient was found to be too ill to withstand the oper-

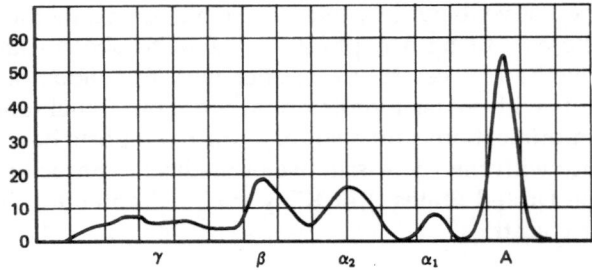

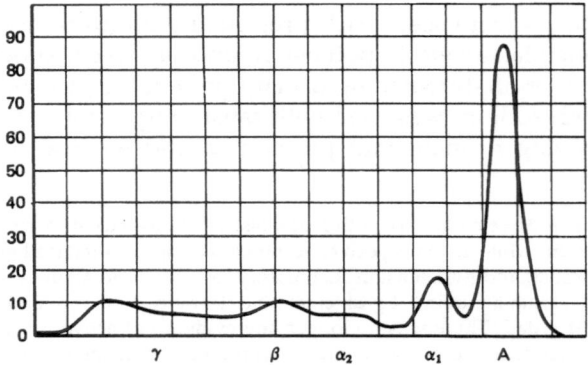

Figure 2. Patterns of serum (top) and urine (bottom) protein electrophoresis in Case 1.

ative procedure. The blood pressure averaged 80/50 mm Hg. The patient was then given a 2-ml solution containing 125 mg of sodium mercaptomerin, equivalent to 40 mg mercury/ml, intramuscularly daily for 6 days. Two days following the last injection, the urinary protein diminished to 4 g/day, and 1 week later the serum albumin was 2.3 g/dl. There was a mild but definite clinical improvement over the next 3 weeks. However, at that time there was a recurrence of massive proteinuria with clinical deterioration. Medical nephrectomy was then repeated with daily mercaptomerin for 10 days, followed by similar improvement. After the second course of therapy, however, the massive proteinuria did not recur. The patient died of a myocardial infarction 2 months following completion of therapy.

Case No. 2. A 49-year-old male was referred with uremia and bilaterally contracted kidneys. An earlier biopsy had shown focal sclerosis. The serum creatinine was 15 mg/dl, creatinine clearance was 4 ml/min, serum complement was normal, and ANA and LE preps were negative. His serum albumin was 1.6 g/dl, and massive low-selectivity proteinuria of 23–30 g/24 h was present.

The patient was treated with hemodialysis with great difficulty because of recurrent hypotensive shock, which occurred with removal of small

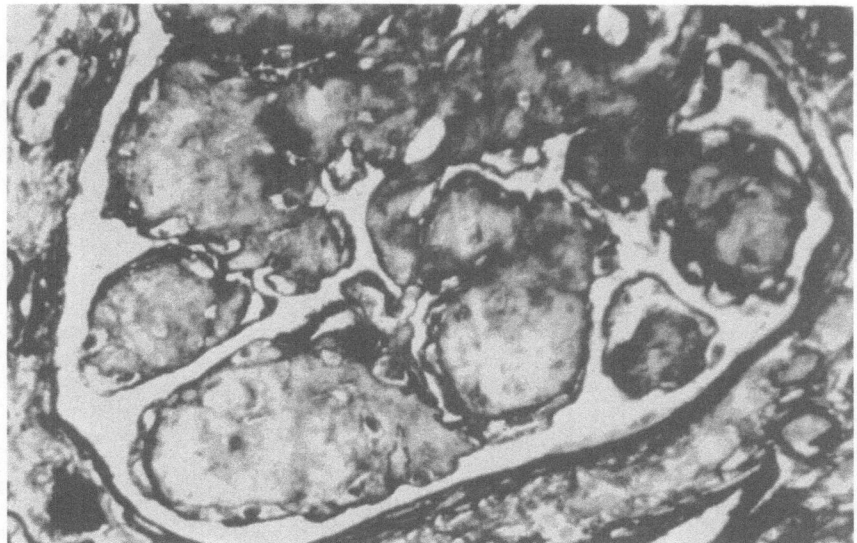

Figure 3. A renal biopsy of Case 1 with PASM stain of a patient with malignant proteinuria, showing large masses of amyloid replacing glomerular lobules. Basement membranes of glomerular tufts (black) outline lubules.

amounts of fluid. Infusions of albumin totaling 300 g during a 2-week period were not sufficient to allow for correction of severe hypotension (85/60 mm Hg) and intravascular volume depletion or to allow for adequate dialysis. Bilateral nephrectomy could not be performed because of the patient's poor condition. Medical nephrectomy was performed in a similar manner as for Case No. 1, following which serum albumin rose to 3.3 g/dl, and urinary protein diminished to 2 g/day. Five weeks following treatment, massive proteinuria recurred, and medical nephrectomy was repeated, with similar improvement in the clinical and laboratory status. Following this, the patient did well for 8 months, at which time a renal transplantation was performed.

In neither of these cases were abnormalities in hematologic, gastrointestinal, cardiac, or neurological systems noted as we watched for mercurially caused symptoms. In spite of careful scrutiny, no gingivitis, stomatitis, diarrhea, tremors, or mental changes were observed.

RESULTS

Following administration of mercurial salts, there was a prompt reduction of urinary output and marked reduction in excreted proteins

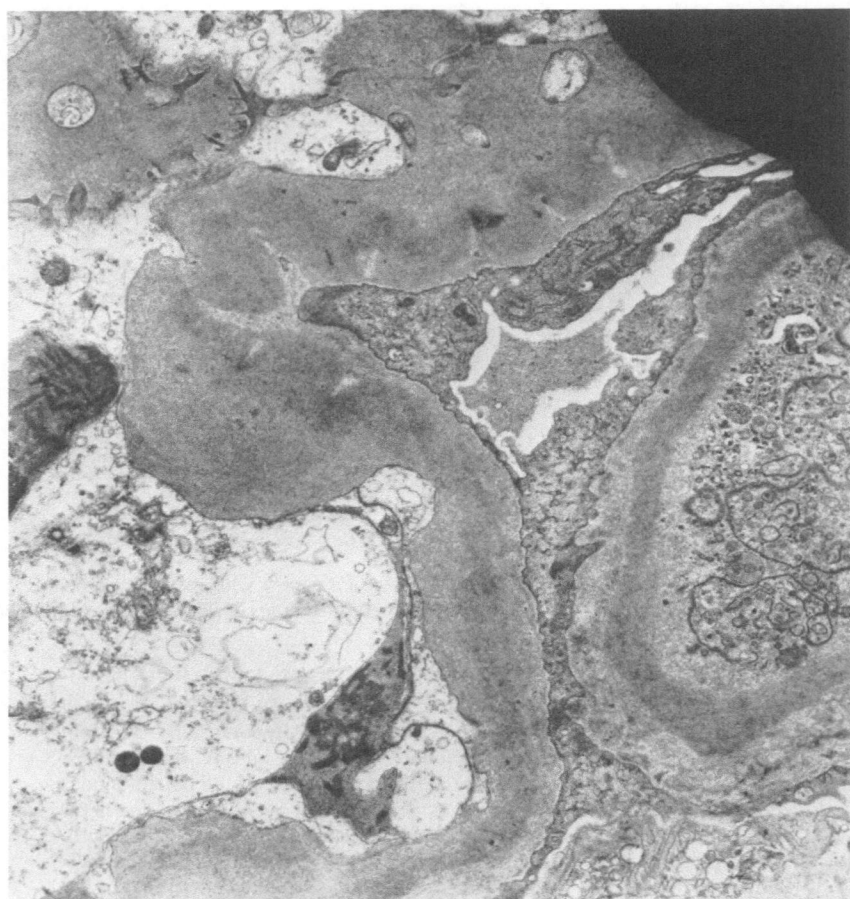

Figure 4. Electron micrograph of amyloid in the glomerulus showing fibrillar structure typical of this nosological entity.

with a gradual rise in serum proteins (Fig. 7). There was a concomitant beneficial rise in systemic blood pressure (80/50 to 125/80 mm Hg in Case No. 1 and 85/60 to 120/75 mm Hg in Case No. 2) to normotensive levels. Effective hemodialysis could now be carried out, the massive edema diminished, and the patients, both previously bed-ridden, could now ambulate without assistance, and life was prolonged. In the period following medical nephrectomy, the hematocrit remained stable, and no

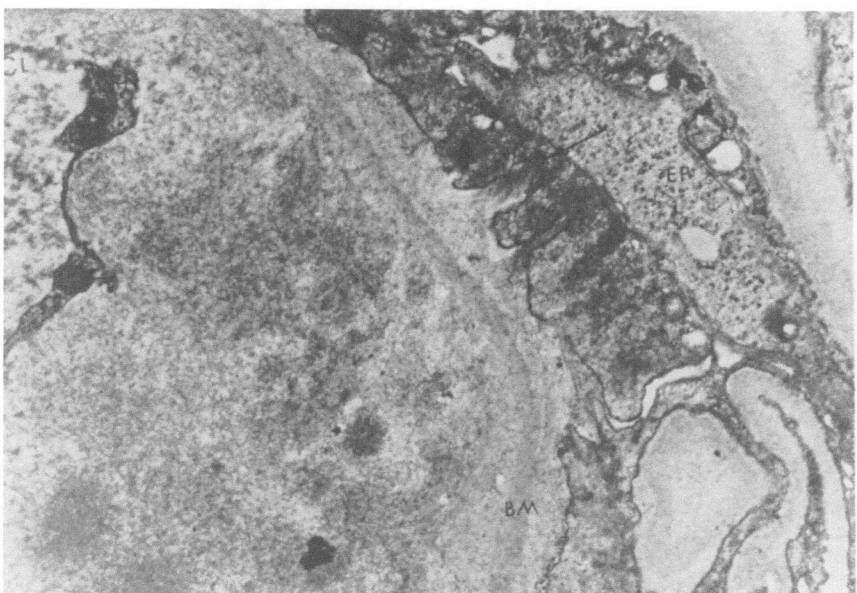

Figure 5. Greater magnification electromicrograph of same amyloid biopsy in which basement membrane and epithelial cell may be seen. BM = basement membrane; EC = epithelial
cell; arrow = pointing at foot processes.

further albumin or blood transfusions were required. No evidence of active bone disease could be detected clinically or by X ray.

The amount of proteinuria in these cases was remarkable in view of
the low glomerular filtration rates. The amount of albumin presented to
the glomeruli in Case No. 1 was:

$$3 \text{ ml/min} \times 1.4 \text{ g/100 ml} \times 1440 \text{ min/day} = 60.5 \text{ g albumin/day}$$

Since about 60% of the urinary protein was albumin, about 30% of the
serum albumin presented to the glomeruli was apparently excreted in
the urine.

Similarly, the amount of albumin presented to the glomeruli in Case
No. 2 was:

$$4 \text{ ml/min} \times 2.1 \text{ g/100 ml} \times 1440 \text{ min/day} = 121 \text{ g albumin/day}$$

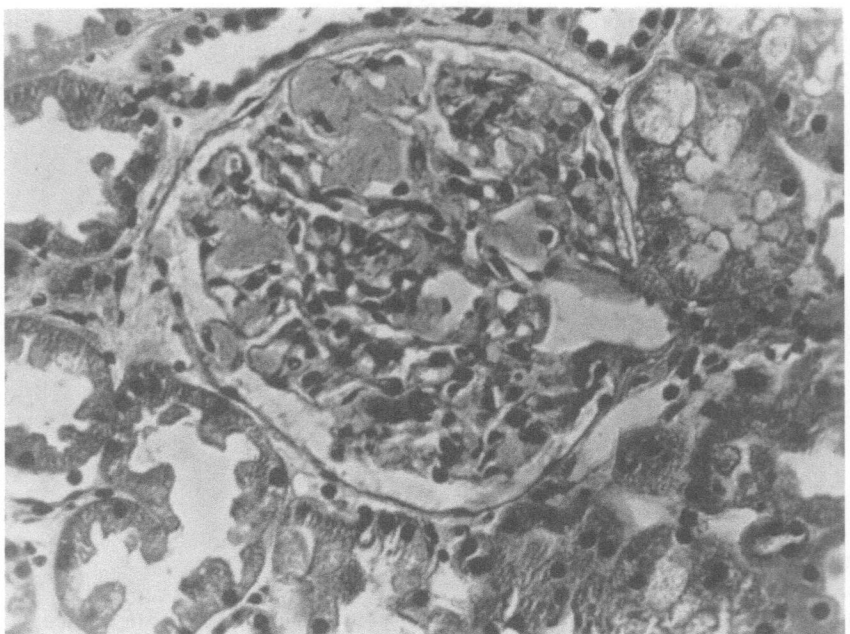

Figure 6. Amyloid in a kidney glomerulus of the type causing massive proteinuria.

Since 60% of the urinary protein was albumin, about 15% of the albumin presented to the glomeruli was excreted. These represent unusually high rates of albumin excretion, and administration of mercurial salts resulted, in each case, in a reversal of this process.

DISCUSSION

The massive proteinuria encountered in some patients is life threatening and this form of nephrotic syndrome sometimes requires extraordinary measures. We have described circumstances that were life threatening and that did, indeed, require extreme therapeutic modalities.

The massive proteinuria in the nephrotic syndrome usually decreases with progression of the renal disease. Failure to decrease urinary loss with decreasing glomerular filtration rate has been noted,[1,2] and it is in this group that the patients' resulting hypoalbuminemia, hypotension, and shock challenge the ingenuity of the nephrologist to devise new therapeutic approaches in order to maintain life.

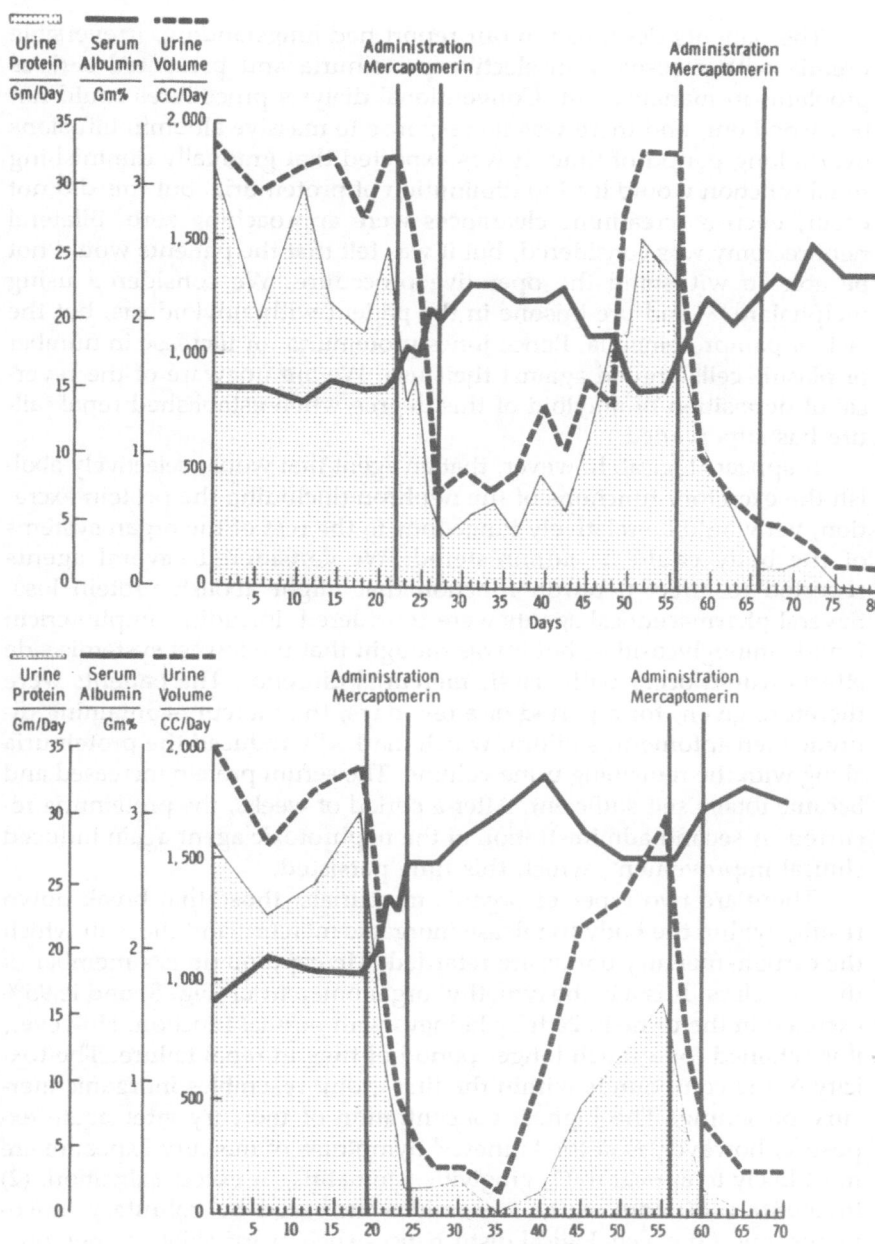

Figure 7. Medical nephrectomy (MN): The use of mercurial salts for reversal of malignant proteinuria (Cases 1 and 2).

The patients described in our report had longstanding, irreversible uremia with massive nonselective proteinuria and presented serious problems in management. Conventional dialysis procedures could not be carried out, and there was no response to massive albumin infusions over a long period of time. It was expected that gradually diminishing renal function would lead to diminution of proteinuria, but this did not occur, even as creatinine clearances were approaching zero. Bilateral nephrectomy was considered, but it was felt that the patients would not be able to withstand the operative procedure. We considered using melphalan[10,11] and prednisone in the patient with amyloidosis, but the lack of paraproteinemia, Bence Jones proteinuria, or increase in number of plasma cells argued against their use. We are unaware of the reversal of deposition of amyloid of this degree when established renal failure has supervened.

It appears logical, however, that an agent that would selectively abolish the excretory functions of the nephron (including the protein excretion) yet would be relatively innocuous to the rest of the organ systems of the body could be administered. We considered several agents reported to affect nephron function that might abolish protein loss. Several pharmaceutical agents were considered, including amphotericin B and aminoglycosides, but it was thought that the fewest systemic side effects would occur with classic mercurial diuretics. The patients were therefore given, for a period of a few days, the mercury-containing diuretic mercaptomerin sodium, which markedly reduced the proteinuria along with the remaining urine volume. The serum protein increased and became totally self-sufficient. After a period of weeks, the proteinuria recurred. A second administration of the nephrotoxic agent again induced clinical improvement, which this time persisted.

There are two types of organic mercurials: those that break down readily within the body to release inorganic mercury and those in which the carbon–mercury bonds are retarded. Mercaptomerin is a member of the first class. It is a carboxymethyl organomercurial (Fig. 8) and is 95% excreted in the urine in 24 h by kidneys with normal function. However, it is retained for a much longer period of time in renal failure. The toxicity of the compounds within the first group resembles inorganic mercury poisoning. The highest concentration of mercury after acute exposure, however, is in the kidney.[12] Symptoms of mercury exposure are most likely to appear in (1) gingivitis, stomatitis, or excess salivation, (2) involuntary tremors of the extremities increased by voluntary movements, and (3) psychological disturbances such as irritability or nervousness. In addition, the heart may show changes of left ventricular hypertrophy. Colic and diarrhea indicate that gastrointestinal dysfunction can also occur.

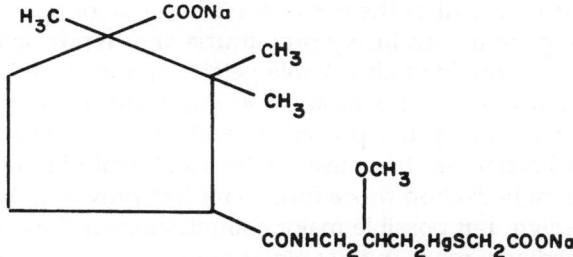

Figure 8. The chemical structure of mercaptomerin sodium.

Mercurial diuretics have been shown to be toxic in the nephrotic syndrome. Schreiner[13] has reported acute tubular necrosis secondary to their use. Mercuric chloride has been used as a model of acute renal failure[14] and has caused renal failure in humans.[15] In these cases, the predominant lesions have been proximal tubule necrosis. Indeed, necrosis in the proximal convoluted tubules and sometimes in the distal tubules has been noted at autopsy.[16] These changes certainly suggest that mercury has caused some damage to the kidney, but tubular lesions alone cannot fully explain the dramatic reduction of protein excretion unless acute tubular necrosis also occurred. Alternatively, another mechanism to explain the diminished proteinuria after a second course of therapy is modification of glomerular basement membrane permeability. A perusal of the literature shows that the glomeruli of patients exposed to mercurial toxins usually appear normal on light microscopy but have not been previously studied with electron microscopy by most authors. However, one case that was normal by light microscopy was found to have dense deposits between visceral epithelial cells on the epithelial side of the basement membrane.[17]

Other renal lesions have been reported in mercury poisoning.[18] Mercurous chloride and ammoniated mercury ointment have been reported to cause nephrotic syndrome, proximal tubular nephropathy, and Fanconi's syndrome.[19] A hypercellular glomerulonephritis has been noted with inorganic mercury compounds.[13] In addition, albuminuria and basement membrane thickening have been described with the absorption of inorganic compounds.[20]

Although no pathological material was available in our cases, the clinical course of reversal after a period of weeks would seem to implicate an initially reversible tubular lesion with reversed acute tubular necrosis, which, after further treatment, became irreversible.

Since our use of mercurial salts, other reports have appeared with other modalities of treatment of massive proteinuria in advanced renal failure. An article describes the use of the technique of renal artery embolization in a patient with heavy proteinuria and hypovolemia. In this case, the authors shredded absorbable gelatin sponge to selectively occlude both renal arteries and produce anuria.[1] The patient developed pain and fever following the procedure and then improved clinically. Selective embolization has been used in the treatment of renal adenocarcinoma.[21] The embolization procedure so far has proved to be relatively simple and benign, but possible major complications include arterial dissection, hemorrhage, reaction to contrast media, and peripheral embolization. This method would appear to be more suited for cases in which complete vascular occlusion is indicated. Also, other reports stress the benefits of unilateral[4] or bilateral nephrectomy[7] for patients with massive intractable proteinuria and progressive complications.

CONCLUSION

Two patients with intractable massive proteinuria and uremia were followed and treated with standard medical therapy and dialysis. After a period of study and demonstration of clinical deterioration, both patients were given solutions containing sodium mercaptomerin. Within days there was a decline in urine protein excretion and a variable increase in serum protein concentration. The patients demonstrated an increase in blood pressure, which made hemodialysis treatment possible. No deleterious effects of the mercury salts were noted. These observations suggest that in selected cases nephrotoxic agents may be of value in decreasing massive proteinuria and improving protein homeostasis in uremic patients.

We describe a new syndrome, which we would like to call "malignant proteinuria," in which over 25g of proteins are lost in the urine in 24 h, with resultant severe hypoproteinemia, edema, and life-threatening hypotension and shock. It is typically present in uremic patients, and these patients have been diagnosed to have focal sclerosis.[1] It can, however, be present in the nonuremic patient, post-transplant, and with only minimal histological changes[5] such as mild increase in mesangial matrix.

For the dialysis-dependent uremic group we describe the use of mercurial salts to effect "medical nephrectomy" with a resultant stop in leakage of proteins, restoration of blood pressure, and preservation of endocrine capabilities of the kidney.

ACKNOWLEDGMENTS. Supported in part by grants from the National Kidney Foundation of New York/New Jersey, Inc. and funds from the

Avram Center for Kidney Diseases of The Long Island College Hospital and a grant from the Nephrology Foundation of Brooklyn.

REFERENCES

1. McCarron DA, Rubin RJ, Barnes BA, et al: Therapeutic bilateral renal infarction in end-stage renal disease. N Engl J Med 294:652, 1976
2. Avram MM, Lipner HL, Gan AC: Medical nephrectomy: The use of metallic salts for the control of massive proteinuria in the nephrotic syndrome. Trans Am Soc Artif Intern Organs 22:431, 1976
3. Montoliu J, Botey A, Torras A, et al: Renin-induced massive proteinuria in man. Clin Nephrol 11:267–271, 1979
4. Shapiro W, Chou SY, Porush JG: Nephrectomy for intractable proteinuria secondary to severe nephrotic syndrome, Abstr Am Soc Nephrol 8:24, 1975
5. McLeish KR, Gohara AF, Shapiro RS: Massive post-transplant proteinuria with minimal histological changes. Transplantation 29:392–396, 1980
6. Payne JE, Silcott GR, Mendez R, et al: Bilateral nephrectomy and renal homotransplantation for malignant nephrosclerosis. Arch Surg 107:17, 1973
7. Aronian JM III, Stubenbord WT, Stenzel KH, et al: Bilateral nephrectomy in chronic hemodialysis and renal transplant patients. Am J Surg 126:634, 1973
8. Rosenberg JC, Azcarate J, Fleischmann LE, et al: Indications for pre-transplant nephrectomy. Arch Surg 107:233, 1973
9. Chrysanthakopoulos SG, Kastagis BK, Jubis W, et al: Hypertension in patients on maintenance hemodialysis: Evaluation of peripheral renin activity and bilateral nephrectomy. Am J Med Sci 264:9, 1972
10. Avram MM, Lipner HI, Huatuco A, et al: Medical nephrectomy—an alternative to surgery in massive proteinuria and malignant hypertension. Cardiovas Med 3:453–458, 1978
11. Kirschbaum BB, Tisnado J: Renal ablation with the Gianturco stainless steel coil for control of massive proteinuria. J Urol 126:807–808, 1981
12. Doolan PD, Hess WC, Kyle LH: Acute renal insufficiency due to bichloride of mercury. N Engl J Med 249:273, 1973
13. Schreiner GE: The nephrotic syndrome, in Straus MB, Welt LG (eds): Diseases of the Kidney. Boston, Little, Brown, 1971, p 600
14. Mandema E, Arends A, Van Zeijst J, et al: Mercury and the kidney. Lancet 1:1266, 1963
15. Riddle M. Gardner F, Beswick I, et al: The nephrotic syndrome complicating mercurial diuretic therapy. Br Med J 1:1274, 1958
16. Kazantzis G: Mercury and the kidney. Trans Soc Occup Med 20:54, 1970
17. Friberg L, Hammarstrom S, Nystram A: Kidney injury after chronic exposure to inorganic mercury. Arch Indust Hyg Occup Med 8:149, 1953
18. Bank N, Mutz BF, Aynedyian HS: The role of "leakage" of tubular fluid in anuria due to mercury poisoning. J Clin Invest 46:695, 1967
19. Becker CG, Becker EL, Maher JF: Nephrotic syndrome after contact with mercury. A report of five cases, three after the use of ammoniated mercury ointment. Arch Intern Med 110:178, 1962
20. Kazantzis G, Scholler KFR, Asscher AW: Albuminuria and the nephrotic syndrome following exposure to mercury and its compounds. Q J Med 31:403, 1962
21. Almgard LE, Fernstrom I, Haverling M: Treatment of renal adenocarcinoma by embolic occlusion of the renal circulation. Br J Urol 45:474, 1973

16

Experience with Medical Nephrectomy

JOHN E. KILEY, GAY CASE, AND JOHN D. BOWER

INTRODUCTION

In the past, patients with nephrotic syndrome have died from severe proteinuria, hypoproteinemia, anasarca, malnutrition, infection, and end-stage renal disease. The development and effective use of more potent diuretics and antibiotics have improved management of these patients, and treatment by dialysis has prevented death when nephrotic syndrome has gone on to end-stage renal failure and uremia. This prevention of death from renal failure and uremia in these patients has also suggested that, if the degree of proteinuria, edema, and malnutrition were life threatening, the patient's life might be saved by altering renal function to decrease proteinuria and then maintaining the patient, if necessary, by chronic dialysis. Reports of ablation of renal function for this purpose have described a number of techniques, including surgical nephrectomy and complete infarction of both kidneys by embolization[1,2] as well as decrease of proteinuria produced either by prostaglandin synthetase inhibitors[3-5] or by administration of metallic salts.[6,7]

This report details a case in which use of a mercuric salt as described by Avram and co-workers was used successfully to perform a virtually complete ablation of kidney function.

CASE REPORT

C.R., a 26-year-old black man, was first referred to the Ward Teaching Service of the University of Mississippi Hospital on September 18, 1980 by his local physician after failure of steroid treatment (80 mg prednisone daily for about 1 month) to improve his nephrotic syndrome. Prior

JOHN E. KILEY, GAY CASE, AND JOHN D. BOWER • Department of Medicine, University of Mississippi Medical Center, Jackson, Mississippi 39216.

to the onset of nephrotic syndrome 2 months previously, the patient had been in good health and worked as a busy cabinet maker. Both of his parents were treated for hypertension, and a grandmother was being treated by hemodialysis in Chicago.

On admission, C.R. was an obese and edematous cushingoid black man of average stature in no acute distress. His blood pressure was 160/90, temperature 98.6°, pulse 80, respirations 18, and weight 90 kg. He showed 4+ pitting edema in the lower extremities and decreased breath sounds with dullness over the bases of both lungs.

Laboratory investigation revealed 4+ protein and many granular casts and oval fat bodies in the urine. His BUN was 31 mg/dl, and serum creatinine was 1.6 mg/dl, serum albumin 1.4 g/dl*, total protein 3.6g/dl, and serum cholesterol 855 mg/dl. Chest X ray was consistent with bilateral pleural effusions. Hematocrit was 37, and white count 11,000 cells/mm^3. There was 13 g of proteinuria per day,* and creatinine clearance was 126 ml/min. Studies to demonstrate an etiology of his nephrotic syndrome were negative.

The patient received a diet limited to 87 mEq of sodium per day with maximal intake of protein of high biological value. On September 24, he had a percutaneous renal biopsy guided by excretory urography. The renal tissue obtained showed only fusion of foot processes and was consistent with lipoid nephrosis. Following the biopsy, the patient had severe acute renal failure necessitating hemodialysis via a Scribner–Quinton shunt until October 10. After dialytic therapy and removal of edema fluid, the patient's weight was reduced to 80 kg. Hospital discharge took place on October 28, 1980, when the serum creatinine ws 4.0 mg/dl.

Nephrologists followed C.R. on an outpatient basis until March 18, 1982. He received a diet limited to 87 mEq of sodium, and protein intake was encouraged. Management of edema required increasing doses of furosemide. A rising blood pressure and serum creatinine led to a clinical diagnosis of focal glomerulosclerosis rather than lipoid nephrosis.

He required readmission to the hospital on March 18, 1982 because of pleurisy, fever, and cough productive of yellow phlegm associated with pneumonia and empyema. At this time, his blood pressure was 140/70; he displayed anasarca and weighed 82 kg. His BUN was 81, serum creatinine 8.2 mg/dl, and serum albumin was 0.9 g/dl. Chest X ray suggested an infiltrate in the right lower lung and bilateral pleural effusions. Sputum examination disclosed sheets of gram-negative pleomorphic coccobacilli, some intracellular, suggesting *Haemophilus influen-*

---

*We employed the MacKay modification of the Shevkey–Stafford method to measure proteinuria and the BCG dye binding method to measure serum albumin.

zae. A right thoracentesis obtained cloudy fluid with 9000 white cells per mm^3, pH 6.9, and an LDH of 1900 versus a plasma LDH of 400 U. Cultures of the pleural fluid grew no organisms. The pneumonia and empyema responded well to treatment by tube drainage of the right pleural cavity and ampicillin and tobramycin, permitting removal of the chest tube on March 24. Nevertheless, anasarca, hypoalbuminemia, malnutrition, and hypotensive episodes persisted and worsened.

Certain details of his further management are displayed in Fig. 1. At this point, he had 35 to 45 g of proteinuria per day. Serum albumin was 0.8mg/dl. Serum creatinine was 7 mg/dl with creatinine clearances ranging from 10 to 15 ml/min. Anorexia, nausea, and vomiting frustrated efforts to give an 87-mEq sodium diet with over 2000 calories and 80 g of protein plus protein supplements. Gradual increase of diuretics to 400 mg of furosemide twice daily, 20 mg of metolazone twice daily, and spironolactone 25 mg four times a day produced sodium excretions ranging from 75 to 281 mEq/day but failed to effect a sustained diuresis. Pro-

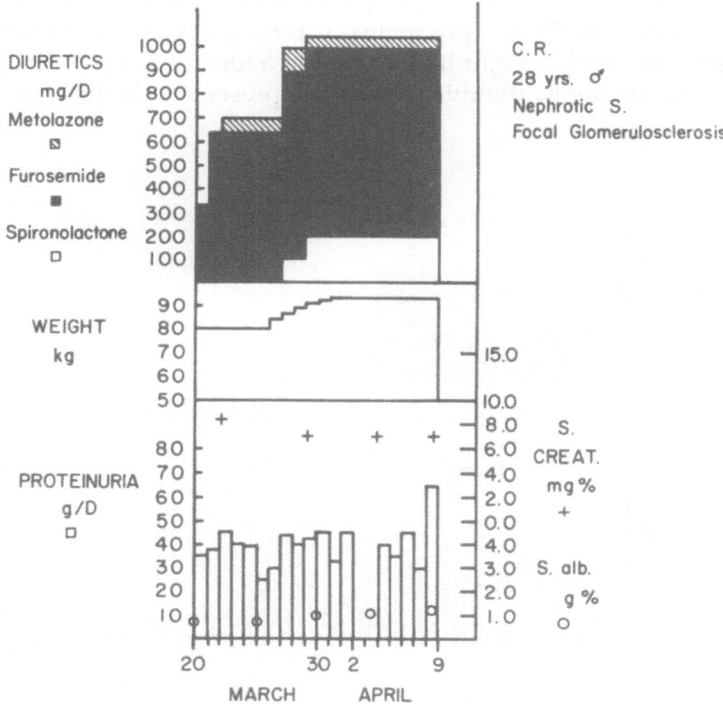

Figure 1. Unsuccessful attempt to effect diuresis.

teinuria rose as high as 65 g/day. The patient left the hospital for an interim period on April 8, 1982.

Further deterioration necessitated readmission on May 1. At this point, the severity of anorexia, nausea, and vomiting and his rate and degree of deterioration compelled us to proceed toward dialysis and medical nephrectomy by injection of a mercuric salt in preference to a trial of indomethacin. Some details of his further course are shown in Fig. 2. At this point, his weight was 100 kg, and serum albumin was 1.0 g/dl. Chronic hemodialysis via Gortex circulation access was begun on May 14, 1982. Despite troublesome hypotensive episodes on dialysis, weight decreased to 85 kg. On May 26, however, because of worsening hypotension during fluid removal, 80 mg of mercury/day was administered intramuscularly via 2 ml of dicurin procaine per day for a 10-day period.

On June 4, the patient transferred to the home training unit, and a dose of 80 mg of mercury per day was given again on June 8, 9, 10, and 11. Urine volume fell to less than a liter a day and by June 25, had decreased to 200 ml with 9.9 g of proteinuria per day. By July 6, 1982, urine volume was 150 ml., proteinuria was 6.5 g/day, and serum albumin had risen to 2 g/dl. Weight had decreased a total of 30 kg to 70 kg, and edema was markedly diminished but still present in the lower extremi-

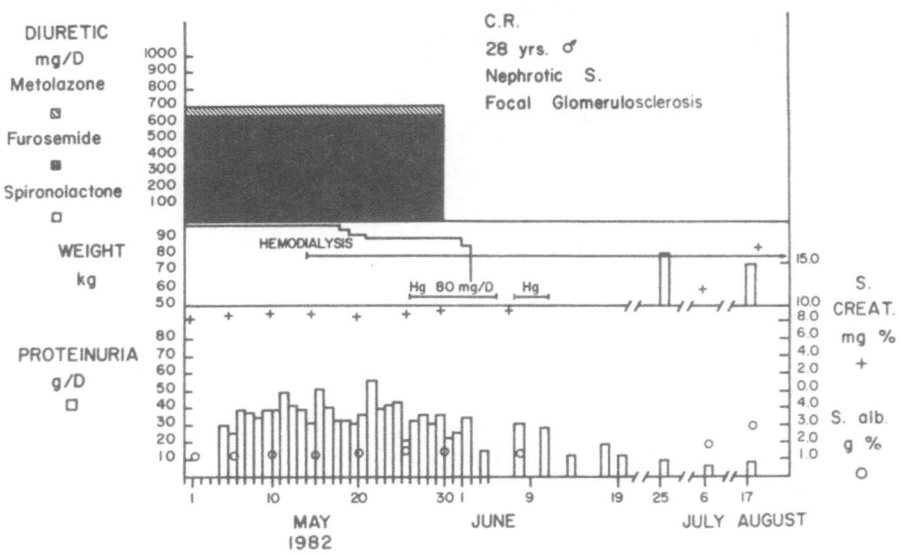

Figure 2. Results of medical nephrectomy.

ties. At this point, hypotension during dialysis no longer posed a problem, and the patient began hemodialysis at home.

By September 7, the patient's weight had decreased to 72.4 kg. His BUN predialysis was 76, and his creatinine 16.6 mg/dl. By November 1, 1982, the patient was free of edema with a weight of 71.5 kg and a serum albumin of 3.7 g/dl. He had a good appetite and was normally active and seeking employment. Predialysis peripheral vein renin was 0.36 ng/ml per h. His urine volumes were 100 to 200 ml/day.

On March 22, 1983, his serum albumin was 4.8 g/dl, and serum cholesterol 165 mg/dl.

DISCUSSION

Our experience with this case treated by mercury injections together with experiences of other members of our staff with treatment by prostaglandin synthetase inhibition or surgical nephrectomy in protein-depleted patients or complete infarction of both kidneys has suggested to us a tentative plan for the management of nephrotic patients whose lives are threatened by massive proteinuria, hypoproteinemia, and severe malnutrition.

We would suggest first a trial of indomethacin to reduce proteinuria and improve serum albumin. The tendency of indomethacin, however, to produce gastrointestinal distress and worsen anorexia, nausea, and vomiting in these patients with consequent poor acceptance and cooperation has occasionally hampered and limited the effectiveness of this approach. In such a situation, we would then proceed to treat these patients by dialysis to reduce edema, bearing in mind that dialysis itself tends to produce a state of oliguria, which may lessen somewhat the degree of proteinuria. Because about 10 g a day of protein is lost in peritoneal dialysate during chronic ambulatory peritoneal dialysis, we prefer hemodialysis to peritoneal dialysis in this situation. If dialysis does not correct the situation, and particularly if the hypoproteinemia is severe enough to make the patient especially liable to severe hypotension and shock during fluid removal, we proceed next to medical nephrectomy. Our tentative protocol is to inject 80 mg of mercury in a mercurial diuretic daily for a period of 10 days as suggested by Avram, followed by a 3- or 4-day interval of no drug administration and then to repeat this procedure as necessary, meanwhile following carefully the total urine volume and protein excretion as well as the state of the gastrointestinal tract, particularly a change in bowel movements toward diarrhea, an indication of the development of colitis from mercury intoxication.

Although medical nephrectomy by salts of mercury or prostaglandin synthetase inhibitors is generally regarded as reversible in its earlier stages, the use of these agents in some patients may be associated with not only complete but also permanent ablation of renal function, particularly when more than one period of administration of mercury salts is employed. This is probably influenced by the fact that patients whose lives are threatened by massive proteinuria, hypoproteinemia, and edema may have severe renal disease that is close to end stage.

The use of bilateral renal infarction by embolization we presently reserve for patients who have not responded adequately to dialysis and medical nephrectomy because of the more invasive nature of the procedures involved and, particularly, difficulties in controlling the degree and localization of embolization as well as the pain and fever often associated with this procedure.

We much prefer to avoid surgical nephrectomy in such seriously protein-depleted patients.

SUMMARY

Consideration of successful use of a mercuric salt for medical nephrectomy in a case of life-threatening nephrotic syndrome, viewed in the light of experience with other techniques for reducing proteinuria in life-threatening nephrotic syndrome, has suggested to us a tentative sequential approach to this type of problem.

ACKNOWLEDGMENTS. The authors wish to express their gratitude to Mrs. C. Fountain for preparation of this manuscript and to Dr. Fred McEwen, Jr. for his help in obtaining dicurin procaine.

REFERENCES

1. Henrich WL, Goldman M, Dotter C, et al: Therapeutic renal arterial occlusion for elimination of proteinuria. *Arch Intern Med* 136:840–847, 1976
2. Thiebot J, Merland JJ, Duboust A, et al: Bilateral nephrectomy by embolization of the renal arteries: A report on five cases. *Sem in Hop Paris* 56:67–675, 1980
3. Donker AJM, Brentjens JRH, van der Hem GK, et al: Treatment of nephrotic syndrome with indomethacin. *Nephron* 22:374–381, 1978

4. Tiggeler RGWL, Hulme B, Wijdeveld PGAB: Effect of indomethacin on glomerular permeability in the nephrotic syndrome. *Kidney Int* 16:312–321, 1979
5. Baumelou A, Legrain M: Medical nephrectomy with anti-inflammatory nonsteroidal drugs. *BR Med J* 284:234, 1982
6. Avram MM, Lipner HI, Gan AC: Medical nephrectomy. The use of metallic salts for the control of massive proteinuria in the nephrotic syndrome. *Trans Am Soc Artif Intern Organs* 22:431–437, 1976
7. Avram MM, Lipner HI: Medical nephrectomy, use of metallic salts as an alternative to bilateral renal infarction. *N Engl J Med* 295:1080, 1976

17

Medical Nephrectomy for Proteinuria

PAUL D. DOOLAN

INTRODUCTION

The problem of large protein loss is one that can take place in many clinical settings. Diabetics, who now constitute a large segment of the American population, are especially prone to develop renal disease and to require some form of maintenance dialysis, either with artificial kidneys or using the peritoneum as a membrane.

CASE HISTORY

We have encountered a patient suffering from diabetes, sepsis pulmonary infiltration, and rising serum creatinine with subsequent massive proteinuria and hypoalbuminemia. In a desperate attempt to prevent this patient's death, we sought to abolish massive protein loss by using medical nephrectomy as described by Avram in this volume (Chapter 15). Others have confirmed the efficacy of medical nephrectomy in the clinical setting (J.E. Kiley et al., Chapter 16, this volume).

We would like to acquaint the reader with the clinical details of this very interesting case. The patient is a 59-year-old insulin-dependent diabetic who was admitted with cellulitis involving the right arm and both legs. He is a reformed alcoholic who in 1972 had an end-to-side portocaval anastomosis. Sepsis, a hemopneumothorax following renal biopsy, a subendocardial infarct, several days of various supraventricular tachycardias, and an additional episode of Staphylococcus aureus bacteremia were the major concerns during the first 64 days of hospitalization. Diffuse bilateral pulmonary infiltrates appeared on day 11 prior to the complications and remained in varying extent and degree through-

PAUL D. DOOLAN • Department of Medicine, Yale University Medical Center, Division of Nephrology, St. Mary's Hospital, Waterbury, Connecticut 06702.

out his hospital stay. The serum creatinine rose gradually over the first 25 days. Periotoneal dialysis was started on day 37 and discontinued on day 62 because of the protein losses in the dialysate up to a high of 9.8 g/exchange, with no evidence of peritonitis.

As the critical problems subsided, attention centered on the inter-related problems of hypoalbuminemia, massive proteinuria, impaired protein synthesis, and postportacaval encephalopathy in this mal-nourished survivor with persistent pulmonary infiltrates interpreted as edema. On day 127 medical nephrectomy was attempted for the follow-ing reasons: the renal biopsy was interpreted as diffuse proliferative glomerulonephritis with active interstitial nephritis consistent with sys-temic vasculitis superimposed on diabetic glomerulopathy. It had been the patient's added misfortune to have progressive renal failure with per-sistent massive proteinuria. He was already on hemodialysis, and it was clear that he would never leave the hospital while requiring daily albu-min infusions, that nutritional rehabilitation was complicated by the al-bumin leak, and that the pulmonary edema was not likely to clear while the plasma colloidal osmotic pressure so easily fell to the 9- to 11-mm Hg range. The pharmacy had no mercurial diuretics, and I had not yet spo-ken with Dr. Avram, so I went ahead with the agent that has gained my respect and resentment, IVP dye: 300 ml 30% diatrizoate was ad-ministered by drip. Predye urine protein loss varied with urine volume from 6 to 24 g/day (28–57 g/liter), and postdye from 4 to 20 g/day (18–31 g/liter). It was considered less than successful, and the patient con-tinued to require albumin infusions.

By day 142 I had spoken to Drs. Avram and Kiley, and indomethi-cin, 50 mg tid, was given for 3 days. The patient's incontinence precluded accurate measurements, but he voided less often, and the im-pression was that the urine volume fell. The decrease was short lived, however, and by days 150 and 151 the protein excretions were 16.4 and 24.6 g/day.

This is a case that is complex, rare, and noteworthy. Complex in the mix and sequence of pathological forces, rare in absolute abstinence from alcohol and 12-year-plus survival post-portocaval anastomosis. It is noteworthy that the IVP dye, indomethicin, and intermittent courses of gentamicin had no lasting effect on the magnitude of the proteinuria (Fig. 1). Whether proteinuria ever warrants the label "malignant" others may be too cautious to allow. Its precision equals that of "medical nephrec-tomy," and I rather like its clarion quality. For those who differ, I hope they allow "perilous," "pernicious," "sinister," or the label of their

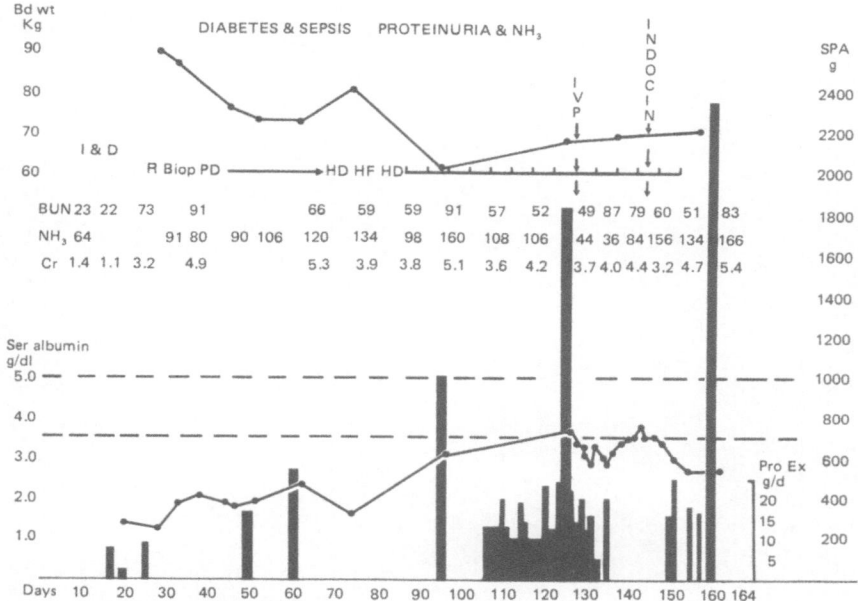

Figure 1. Attempted medical nephrectomy with IVP dye and indomethacin in a diabetic who also received intermittent gentamicin.

choice, because there are such cases. They deserve thoughtful consideration for noninvasive suppression of excretory function, and Dr. Avram has done a service in recommending that we study the problem further.

Epilogue

RICHARD J. GLASSOCK

We have been treated to a potpourri of expositions around the central theme: the appearance of plasma proteins in the urine. These included, according to the bridal aphorism, "something new, something old, something borrowed," but nothing blue.

My general impressions of the conclusions that may be derived from the contributions to this volume are (1) that we now have at hand methods to better understand the mechanisms of and, therefore, to more appropriately classify the various forms of abnormal proteinuria; (2) that we have a better appreciation of some of the clinical consequences of proteinuria; and (3) that much more work needs to be done to bring the fruits of this new understanding to the clinical sphere. Very exciting and exceedingly worthy of further exploration are the new concepts of the conversion of a negatively charged isoporous glomerular capillary wall to a neutral heteroporous capillary wall as glomerular disease progresses.

It would appear that both qualitative and quantitative assays of urinary proteins are useful tools for the detection of glomerular and tubular proteinuria and the assessment of the nature of the underlying abnormality. However, we should not neglect the possible role of abnormal glomerular permeability itself as a cause of progressive renal failure. For example, it could be postulated that the breakdown of the endothelial cell–glomerular basement membrane barrier would expose the glomerular epithelial cells to a very abnormal milieu of a protein-rich fluid, which could exert a pathogenic effect such as the loss of filtration slits and reduced filtering surface area. Furthermore, interaction of the filtered protein with Tamm–Horsfall protein at the level of the ascending limb of the loop of Henle, forming occlusive casts, may result in a deterioration in glomerular filtration rate. The loss of serum albumin, antiplatelet aggregatory factors, antithrombin, and antiplasmin and abnormal lipid bi-

RICHARD J. GLASSOCK • Department of Medicine, UCLA School of Medicine, Harbor-UCLA Medical Center, Torrance and Los Angeles, California 90024.

osynthesis and metabolism could also lead to intracapillary platelet aggregation, fibrin thrombi, and inefficient removal of spontaneously formed fibrin strands, thus leading to intracapillary luminal occlusion from repeated thrombosis. Release of platelet-derived growth factors from such platelet aggregates could also lead to the abnormalities of mesangial cell proliferation. Thus, nephrotic states may have self-perpetuating features. If these postulated phenomena are real, then early aggressive management designed to reduce the magnitude of, rather than to eliminate, proteinuria may be indicated.

Renal biopsy, despite the recent clamor to diminish its clinical value in therapeutic decision making in patients with idiopathic nephrotic syndrome, remains, in my opinion, a useful tool in the assessment of potential responsiveness of proteinuric states and in deciding the vigor with which one would pursue pharmacological management.

We are still forced to lump together pathogenetically heterogeneous disorders under single headings based on crude tools such as light microscopy, immunofluorescence, and electron microscopy. These techniques are clearly insufficient to make the fine-tuned assessment of uniformity of disease. The nonspecificity of focal and segmental glomerular sclerosis with respect to underlying pathogenesis can be cited as a classic example. Focal and segmental glomerular sclerosis is not a disease but a descriptive pathological term. It is a pattern of response to a variety of injurious events. Prompt recurrence of nephrotic proteinuria in renal allografts of some patients with focal and segmental glomerular sclerosis and our inability thus far to identify a circulating factor responsible for the abnormal proteinuria are a potent reminder of our ignorance of the pathogenesis of nephrotic-range proteinuria. Malignant proteinuria and medical nephrectomy are interesting observations.

Although I certainly agree that head-out water immersion has no immediate therapeutic value, I would conclude that the technique has some relevance to the current debate as to whether renal sodium retention in nephrotic syndrom is secondary to an underfilled circulation or whether sodium retention in nephrotic states is a primary intrarenal event associated with or causing an overfilled circulation. The dramatic natriuresis with increased osmolar clearance and improving free water clearance could be used as an argument in favor of the underfilled circulation with secondary antidiuretic hormone release and enhanced sympathetic activity.

Thus, as is the case with many published manuscripts, we find that great strides have been made in basic understanding of the processes responsible for abnormal proteinuria. Real progress in translating these advances to the bedside have been slow to occur. Little change in our empirical treatment of nephrotic syndrome has occurred in the last decade. However, with this new knowledge and a clearer idea of the critical questions that need resolution, we can hope that the next Long Island College Hospital Symposium on Proteinuria will give the clinician some new tools to use in preventing or alleviating the morbidity and mortality associated with the proteinuric disorders.

Index